Jasper County Public Library System

Overdue notices are a courtesy of
the library system.
Failure to receive an overdue notice
does not absolve the borrower of the
obligation to return materials on time.

ANSWERS
TO FREQUENTLY ASKED QUESTIONS
IN PARKINSON'S DISEASE

A RESOURCE BOOK

FOR PATIENTS AND FAMILIES

DAVID L. CRAM, M.D.

Acorn Publishing
A Division of Development Initiatives

Answers to Frequently Asked Questions in Parkinson's Disease
© 2001 David L. Cram, M.D.

Acorn Publishing
A Division of Development Initiatives
P.O. Box 84
Battle Creek, MI 49016-0084

Printed in the United States of America
First Edition, 2002

The images used herein © 2000-2002 www.arttoday.com.

Library of Congress Cataloging-in-Publication Data

Cram, David L. (David Lee), 1934-
  Answers to frequently asked questions in parkinson's disease : a
resource book for patients and families / David L. Cram, M.D.-- 1st ed.
     p. cm.
Includes bibliographical references and index.
  ISBN 0-9710988-8-3
  1. Parkinson's disease--Popular works. I. Title.
  RC382 .C915 2002
  616.8'33--dc21
                              2002001074

The treatment and results the author has experienced may not be similar to that found by other doctors or their patients with this disease. The author's experience with therapy came as a result of the advice of his neurologist. This book is not intended to be advice from the author that is contrary to or serves as a substitute for an attending physician.

ISBN 0-9710988-8-3

A portion of the proceeds from the sale of this book will
go to The National Parkinson Foundation, Inc.

For current information about all releases by Acorn Publishing,
visit our web site: http://www.acornpublishing.com

CONTENTS

FOREWORD

As medicine becomes more sophisticated and technical, physicians have found it harder to keep pace with new developments in their field. Moreover, the increasing and often conflicting demands on physicians' time have made them less available to answer questions that patients may have about their disease. This is true in Parkinson's Disease (PD) where, because of time restraints, important questions may go unanswered. Where then can PD patients and their families turn for these answers?

A good example of where to turn is to the internet where Dr. David Cram has taken on the task of reaching out to patients with PD with answers to many of their questions. Dr. Cram was a very successful dermatologist to whom patients came from all over the country for advise before he was stricken by PD and could no longer practice. The transition from physician to patient was not easy for him, but he has seized the opportunity, in the face of adversity, to fulfill an important need; serving as an intermediary between the medical profession on the one hand, and patients and their families on the other. Through his e-mail column on Age Net, patients have turned to him with their fears, hopes, and questions. His replies have been in a positive vein, allaying concerns, suggesting solutions, providing information, and dispensing advice designed to help patients and their families come to terms with a disease that can be physically and emotionally overwhelming. He has not hesitated to refer to his own difficulties with PD in advising others who face similar problems. At the same time he has used his medical background to gain significant knowledge about PD, which he consistently conveys in language that is easily understood.

Dr. Cram's blend of humanism and professionalism makes this new book remarkable. Patients and their families will gain new knowledge and comfort from reading this book, as it provides sound practical advice and background information about PD and its most up-to-date treatments and discoveries.

During his active professional life Dr. Cram was recognized by patients for his warmth, understanding, and kindness. This book brings these qualities to a much wider public, while at the same time providing an informational resource that will be widely appreciated.

I feel privileged in being able to introduce this book. As Director of the Parkinson's Disease Clinic at the University of California Medical Center in San Francisco, I treat many hundreds of PD patients. I believe that patients everywhere will benefit from reading this book. Indeed, it is also my belief that many healthcare professionals, physicians, nurses, physical therapists, occupational therapists, and other paramedical personnel, will also benefit from the insight that Dr. Cram provides into PD and its impact on the daily lives of patients.

Michael J. Aminoff, M.D., D.Sc.
Professor of Neurology
University of California, San Francisco

"I became convinced that creativity, the will to live, hope, faith, and love have biochemical significance and contribute strongly to healing and to well being."

Norman Cousins

Anatomy of an Illness

INTRODUCTION

Parkinson's disease (PD) affects one million Americans with 50,000 new cases diagnosed each year. The disease can attack anyone, at almost any age and in any walk of life—including celebrities. The recognition of PD affecting a popular American actor less than forty years of age was a shocking reminder that PD is not exclusively a disease of old age. His announcement rekindled the public's interest and brought us a new awareness of the magnitude of the problem. It now seems that everywhere we turn, we learn of someone new who has PD. With so many people suffering worldwide, it is urgent that we not only have governmental support for research activities, but that we find ways to raise the considerable moneys that are needed for the exciting ongoing research that could bring us a cure in this decade.

For those of us who suffer with PD, a cure can not come any too soon. Until that time comes, however, we need to know more about the disease and learn the best ways to cope with its progressive nature. I am convinced that the more I have learned about PD and its course, the better I have come to accept it; that alone has improved the quality of my life.

In early 1999, after having had PD for ten years, and learning as much as I could about it, I wrote a book entitled: ***Understanding Parkinson's Disease. A Self-Help Guide***. This book was the result of my search for a better life with PD. At about the same time, Age Net, an internet service promoted primarily to the elderly, created a web site for me and asked that I start an e-mail question column. My contribution to this column has been to accept questions about PD from interested readers and answer those for which I could give a practical answer. I have made it clear that I am a retired dermatologist, not a neurologist, and I don't attempt to answer technical questions best left to a neurological specialist.

From my active web site I have accumulated a considerable file of commonly asked questions about PD. These are followed by carefully worded answers, some of which include my personal experiences. Since none of this correspondence has ever been made available to the public, I would like to share with you some of the frequently asked questions that have come from medical professionals, patients, family members, caregivers and others interested in PD. (The names have been changed to protect confidentiality.) In addition, following many of the e-mail questions and answers, I have included a concise, up-to-date review of the subjects in question, as well as the results of any new research. I will also try to dispel some of the myths and misconceptions surrounding the disease.

The organization and contents of this book are such that it can be used as an easy-to-read resource book for information on PD. By looking in the Table of Contents one can selectively find the subject of interest and go directly to it. Once there, you will learn more about symptoms, suggested strategies for addressing them, the overall principles of management, the expected results, and any promising research.

It is my hope that the sharing of in-depth information, as well as the inclusion of my own personal experiences with PD, will provide patients and their families with the inspiration, confidence, and knowledge needed to better cope with this distressing disease.

David L. Cram, M.D.

1

Financial Considerations

Where to Turn for Help

A diagnosis of PD can have a devastating effect on the finances of some patients and their families. We know that many people with PD are diagnosed over the age of sixty. They are often close to retirement age, have usually secured their retirement nest egg, and may choose to quit working. On the other hand, younger individuals, especially if they are the family bread-winner, face a new set of questions:

- Can I continue to work?
- For how long will I be able to work?
- Can I be fired from my job?
- Where can I turn for help?

To continue working and for how long depend on what type of work you do and the severity of your PD. Obviously, if you are a brain surgeon you will need to quit as soon as possible. For jobs requiring much less dexterity and skill, you may be able to continue working and this should be encouraged. Your doctor should be able to help you with these kind of decisions. There is a general misconception that once you are diagnosed with PD you must quit working. Many people remain vital and active for years in the same occupation, profession, or place of employment. Also remember, PD is a disability, protected by federal law which means you cannot be fired on account of it. If this becomes an issue, it may, however, prove costly to win such a case in court.

If finances are a problem, where can one turn for help? Many PD patients have written to me about this problem as in the question that follows.

QUESTION:

Dear Dr. Cram,

My husband has had early onset PD for over fourteen years. We recently moved into a condominium to be near our children. To complicate matters I had a ruptured aneurysm thirteen years ago, which affected my short term memory—so much so that I have trouble coping with daily living. My daughter and her husband have been questioning my ability to continue my care for my husband, as they also see more of his escapades. He can not be left alone, cannot dress himself or perform any of the daily things necessary including personal grooming, I suppose my question is: At what point do I give up on taking care of him by myself? Is there a way to pay for good care on a limited income? Thank you for your time.

ANSWER:

Betty, your heart-breaking story is like so many I receive where PD has not only destroyed the patient's life, but has left the family in difficult financial straits. Bless your heart for your devotion to your husband, despite your own difficulties. Exploring the resources that might be available to you can be difficult, because they vary from state to state. Some services are only available in large metropolitan centers. My answer follows:

First of all, your daughter and her husband are right. With your disability and failing memory you are not in a position to properly care for your husband much longer. So, what are some of your options?

- Your husband should be receiving Social Security and Medicare, since he has been disabled for more than two years. Phone Medicare and find out what else might be available for your husband. Medicare is listed in your phone book.

- Also ask about Medicaid. Medicare will not cover nursing home fees or the cost of an Alternative Care Facility, but Medicaid will if your financial situation meets the requirements. Medicare can also provide only limited home care services

- To qualify for Medicaid you must have a low income and limited resources. You should consider Medicaid carefully, as it may not be in your best interests and there may be other alternatives. You might, for example, be able to join an HMO. Your doctor or a social worker should be able to help you decide.

7

- Some states have "insurance pools" available for those people who meet certain requirements. To find out about this service contact your state or local legal aid society by looking in the yellow pages of the phone book. Many law schools may also provide such low or no cost legal and financial services.

- You may be able, by calling a Legal Aid or Consumer Crediting Counseling, to receive help on how to manage your financial situation. This could be at no cost, if you meet certain requirements.

- Check your state's Area Office on Aging for a list of services offered in your community. Check your local phone book for their number as well as subjects listed under "Community Services" and "Senior Services." These are usually found in the telephone book's yellow pages. Along the way, as you explore these options, you should learn more about other areas of aid best suited for your husband, based on your available income.

- Unfortunately, it sounds like your husband may very soon need nursing home care. Your doctor and a social worker should be able to help you here. A qualified social worker can be found through your doctor, a local hospital, or a registered nurse. If you have no medical insurance, a social worker can often help you obtain affordable coverage and advise you in seeking further care. I also suggest you call or write: The American Parkinson Disease Association Inc., 1250 Hylan Blvd., Suite 48, Staten Island, N Y 10305 (800-223-3732) for a copy of "The

Challenge of Parkinson's Disease: Adapting To A Nursing Home" by Karla Tolson. This brief article can help you in your decision or at least give you a better feel for what you will be dealing with. Also see the valuable section on Resources at the end of this book. Don't get discouraged, as help is available.

STAYING IN THE WORK FORCE

Most people, after being diagnosed with PD, begin to worry about what they will do now that they have the disease. Some are happy to retire, but most want to be busy, despite any limiting symptoms. The following is an e-mail from a concerned daughter worried about her mother's reduced financial opportunities and about ways to keep her active.

QUESTION:

Dear Dr. Cram,

Thank you for your informative and honest expression about your experience with PD. My mother has been diagnosed with PD and I am very concerned watching as financial opportunities in business had to change due to her disease. I am now realizing that she has to think about new ways to keep herself active that are not like the demanding and competitive marketplace. Thank you for your insight.

ANSWER:

Thank you, Susan, for your kind remarks. As regards your mother and her options, I firmly believe that all PD patients should try to remain in the work force as long as possible. This is especially true in early onset PD. It is important not only for monetary reasons, but it helps preserve one's self-esteem. I don't know what your mother did before she had PD, but if there is a way she could work out of her home, using a computer, a fax, and a telephone, she could remain in the work force for several years depending on the severity of her PD. If this is not possible, remember we all have hidden talents that we should consider. For me, it turned out to be writing. For others, it might be gourmet cooking, gardening, photography, learning the computer, teaching a class out of your home, or volunteer work. In addition, with her doctor's permission, one of the most important steps your mother could take to preserving her health is to establish an exercise program. Encourage her to learn all she can about PD, remember to take her medications on time, stay active in her community, place of worship, and with a circle of friends. Let her be as independent as she can for as long as she can. And tell her never to give up hope. The future for PD patients looks bright. Thank you for your question and good luck to your mother.

2

DIAGNOSING EARLY DISEASE AND TREMOR

EARLY STAGES OF PARKINSON'S DISEASE

One of the most frequently asked questions I receive is: "How is the diagnosis of PD made?" Wondering if they have PD, people often write in describing early subtle symptoms.

PD can be a difficult disease to diagnose—especially in its early stages. Unfortunately, at this time there are no laboratory tests or x-rays that help. The following are examples of the kind of questions I receive about early PD:

QUESTIONS:

• *Exactly how is PD diagnosed? Are there any specific tests that confirm that you have it? My symptom is tremor in my hands and slight tremor of my jaw. The tremor is particularly bothersome when I am trying to do needlework, etc.*

• *I am a fifty year old woman and I am wondering if I might have PD. Last week while I was showering I looked at my hands and found the ring and little fingers trembling. It seems to be more pronounced*

in the shower and slight to faint during the day.
Sometimes I feel that my speech is thick, but this is
infrequent. I feel some muscle stiffness, but figure
that is the effects of old age. Any suggestions?

• *I have been told by a neurologist that I have parkin-*
sonism. Comparing classic PD symptoms with mine,
I find I match rather closely except for having very
little tremor. It is not pronounced and not constant.
Usually occurs when eating or playing cards. I am
confused. Do I have PD or not? If yes, what further
should be done?

• *My mother has been diagnosed with PD. The only*
symptom that seems to be mentioned in all cases is
tremor. This is the one thing she does not have. I
would like to know if this is always present? She
does speak in a very soft tone. She loses her train
of thought. She appears to have a form of dementia
in that she can not remember events that happened
in the past. What are some of the symptoms that aid
in the diagnosis? Are there tests to determine PD?

ANSWER:

PD can be difficult to diagnose in its early stage even
by the best neurologists. The diagnosis is based largely on
four physical findings, especially the type of tremor. One
common misconception is that all tremors are due to PD.
This is not so. Tremors can be hereditary as in essential
tremor, secondary to alcohol abuse, occur following caffeine and nicotine withdrawal, and in thyroid disease—
just to mention a few. To add to the diagnostic dilemma,
statistics reveal that 30 percent of PD patients have no

significant tremor. The diagnosis must then hinge on the other diagnostic symptoms. The four diagnostic findings useful in making the diagnosis of PD are:

☞ **Tremor at rest** - tremor that disappears as we move the affected part.

☞ **Slowness of movement** - the affected person may not even be aware of this and it is noticed first by a spouse or friend. This often produces a shuffling gait.

☞ **Stiffness and rigidity of muscles.**

☞ **Unstable balance and lack of coordination.**

Not all of these features are required to make a clinical diagnosis. At an early stage only one or two may be present. Tremor is the first manifestation in most cases and neurological examination is important to distinguish it from other causes of tremor. Some might add to this list a positive response to a trial of levodopa (Sinemet), a common drug used in treating PD. Some neurologists warn that this kind of test can be unreliable and confuse the clinician. A positive family history of PD also helps; only rarely, however, is a family history present.

By now, you have heard the word *"Parkinsonism."* What does it mean? Parkinsonism is a general term applied to patients who present with the four diagnostic symptoms listed above, but do not necessarily have typical, idiopathic PD. These same four symptoms can be produced by other causes, such as certain drugs, toxins and blows to the head, and even a stroke, just to mention a few. With a negative history for other possible causes, is typical PD then the considered diagnosis? Not completely. There are several other rare neurological conditions, that mimic typical PD, so called "Atypical PD" or "Parkinson's-Plus," that can be hard to differentiate. These rare conditions can be difficult to diagnose and may require an MRI or other sophisticated tests. It sometimes takes a long period of observation to properly identify these other diseases.

There is a method for the detection of PD, as reported in a review article in the July, 1999 issue of the *Mayo Clinic Proceedings*. Mayo Clinic researchers reported on a technique that appears to determine the status of dopamine-producing neurons in the substantia nigra of the brain. The discovery uses a widely available brain imaging technique called Single-Photon Emission Computer Tomography (SPECT) in combination with the injected investigational drug called beta CIT. This drug, beta CIT, when injected into the blood stream, binds selectively to dopaminergic nerve cells in the brain. After the drug is given, the SPECT camera is able to measure how much of the drug binds to the neurons. Using this technique the Mayo researchers were able to differentiate between ten PD patients and ten normal controls. The drug detected in the PD group was reduced. They also studied ten blood relatives of PD patients and found that the amount of drug bound to the nerve cells was in a range between that of the PD patients and the normal controls.

The goal of this research is to try to determine who is at risk of developing PD and to identify therapies that can delay or even prevent the onset of the disease in high risk individuals. If these imaging findings are confirmed, quantified, and proven to be a consistent finding, doctors will have a technique to help confirm the diagnosis of PD. Perhaps of even greater importance is that this may prove to be a method to detect this crippling disease well before full blown signs and symptoms appear. If proven correct the next step would be to try and delay or even prevent the onset of the disease in these people. Eventually this technique may become commonplace for the diagnosis of PD, but how soon this will be is unknown.

For now, the only way to be sure you have PD when you have suspicious or subtle symptoms is to get a neurological exam, preferably done by a neurologist with a special interest in PD. Sometimes in very early PD the doctor will have to advise watchful waiting until the disease progresses and the diagnosis becomes clear. This may take two or three years in some cases.

References:

Calne, D. B., Snow, B. J., and Lee, C. 1992. "Criteria For Diagnosing Parkinson's Disease." *Annals of Neurology.* 32:125-127

Hoehm, M. M., and Yahr, M. D. 1967. "Parkinsonism: Onset, Progression and Mortality." *Neurology.* 17:427-442.

Marck, K. L., Scibyl J., Zoghbi S.S. et al. 1996. "B-CIT/SPECT Imaging Demonstrates Bilateral

Loss of Dopamine Transporters in Hemi-Parkinson's Disease." *Neurology.* 46:231-237

YOUNG-ONSET PARKINSON'S DISEASE

One of the most common misconceptions, recently dispelled, is that PD is a disease of old age. We think of the disease as a stereotype of an old, stooped and tremulous person. PD can start at almost any age, even in children—although this is extremely rare, except in Japan. In that country onset of PD before age twenty-one is common. The announcement by the young American actor, Michael J. Fox, that he has PD was a revelation that sparked new insight and interest in the disease. Several people asked for more information on Young-Onset PD (YOPD).

QUESTION:

Dear Dr. Cram,

It is said that Michael J. Fox, the actor, has early onset PD. I guess it started in his thirties. How is his PD different from the usual disease seen in older people? Watching him on TV, he seems to be getting worse, showing signs of unusual head and face movements. I really enjoy his show. My father had PD, but his started at about age sixty I am fairly sure. He never had movements like that. In fact, he had little tremor except when under stress. Thank you for your column.

ANSWER:

Dear Al,

Young-onset (or early onset) PD is defined as PD with motor symptoms beginning before age forty. The average age of onset of typical PD is approximately sixty-two. However, between five and ten percent of patients report the onset of PD before the age of forty. In recent years researchers have turned their attention to the YOPD which appears between the ages of twenty-one and forty. Cases that develop before age twenty-one are called Juvenile Parkinsonism (JP) or Parkinson's Syndrome, as they appear to be a mix of conditions and will not be discussed.

There are some differences between late onset PD and YOPD. Although the early symptoms are similar, YOPD progresses more slowly than late onset PD. YOPD tends to respond even better to levodopa, but distressing side effects from this drug, especially dyskinesias, tend to appear earlier in treatment of YOPD. In fact, they may appear within a few months of starting levodopa.

There is now new evidence that genetics may play a significant role in this younger onset disease. YOPD patients are more likely to report relatives with PD. There is also a higher rate of depression in YOPD.

A few years ago some Japanese scientists discovered a rare form of early onset PD called Autosomal Recessive-Juvenile PD. They searched for a gene that might cause this form of early onset PD and they found it. They called it the Parkin gene. Published reports now show the Parkin gene is associated with PD throughout the world. Although most PD patients do not have this gene, at least 25 percent of people with early onset PD have the abnormal Parkin gene. Some have even considered, because of this finding, that YOPD may prove to be a different disease.

Because YOPD tends to respond well to levodopa and the disease progression is slow, the patient should stay in the work force until it becomes too difficult to continue. This is what I understand Mr. Fox plans to do. That will benefit all of us who enjoy his talent.

References

Golbe, L. I., "Young-Onset Parkinson's Disease: A Clinical Review." 1991. *Neurology.* 41:168-173

Cimons, M., "Sufferers Find Parkinson's is No Respecter of Youth." *Los Angeles Times.* August 4, 1991

Golbe, L. I. 1993. "Risk Factors In Young-Onset Parkinson's Disease." *Neurology.* 43:1641-1643.

Ishikawa, A., Tsuji, S. 1996. "Clinical Analysis of 17 Patients In 12 Japanese Families With Autosomal Recessive Type Juvenile Parkinsonism." *Neurology.* 47:160-166

Kitada, T., Asakawa, S., Hattori, N. et al. 1998. "Mutations In The Parkin Gene Cause Autosomal Recessive Juvenile Parkinsonism." *Nature.* 392:605-608.

ESSENTIAL TREMOR

Essential tremor (familial tremor) is the most common of the neurological movement disorders. Estimates are that essential tremor (ET) is five to ten times more frequent than PD. Since it can resemble PD, especially in early stages, it has been misdiagnosed as PD. One misconception is that ET is at the end of a spectrum of PD—implying that they are the same disease.

QUESTION:

Dear Doctor Cram,

I have essential tremor. My physician has said that this is the other end of the spectrum from PD. What does this mean? I do have problems with my hands and precise work is almost impossible. Also holding large items becomes difficult. I have recently noted a head bobbing that causes me some problems. I am taking Atenolol three times a day. This appears to be most helpful. What other things can I expect?

ANSWER:

Dear Robyn,

Essential tremor is something we older people grew up with, as we watched it slowly progress in one of the great actresses of this century, Katharine Hepburn. We watched over the years as her head bobbing and shaking voice got worse. But her life went on; her acting only got better despite her condition; playing tennis had been her favorite pastime. She is now ninety-four.

One common misconception is that Katharine Hepburn has PD. She has ET. Another misconception is that ET is at the end of a spectrum of PD. ET and PD are separate diseases. On rare occasions people with ET may also develop PD; in other words, the patient has both diseases. This should be anticipated, as they are both relatively common neurological disorders.

Because symptoms of ET can be mild, many patients never consult a physician. The word essential means there is no associated disease or known cause. ET is characterized by onset at any age, but usually in middle life, as an involuntary, rhythmic tremor of a body part, usually the hands and arms. It most commonly is a slowly progressive disease, which eventually may involve the head, voice, tongue, legs and trunk. ET is rarely disabling. In some people it never progresses and only a mild tremor remains for life. Genetics plays a role as almost half of the cases run in families. In familial cases, the inheritance is autosomal dominant, meaning that half the children of the affected may develop the disease.

Distinguishing ET from PD is usually straightforward. There are clear diagnostic differences between the two conditions.

- First of all, the tremor is different. ET tremor occurs with activity, PD tremor occurs at rest.

- The tremor of PD does not involve the head (but it may affect the lower lip or jaw). ET tremor does.

- ET tremor tends to be bilateral (both sides) whereas in PD it is more on one side than the other.

- ET tremors are absent during sleep; mild PD tremors can be present during sleep although are usually absent.

- People with ET also may have a tremor demonstrated by having the patient hold out their outstretched hands (postural tremor) or tremor brought on by voluntary actions such as picking up a glass of water (action tremor).

As ET progresses the patient may rarely develop varying degrees of functional disability. They may have difficulty performing tasks such as holding or manipulating small objects, writing—which with ET may be large, scrawled, and wavy—eating, applying makeup, shaving, and even dressing.

The next part of the body to eventually be involved in ET is the head; in some cases ET may begin in the head. Here the tremor of the head, like the hands, helps in the diagnosis it is so typical. It is rapid and constant. It is either in a horizontal plane, so called "no-no" pattern (75 percent start this way) or in a vertical "yes-yes" pattern. Over time changes in the voice can lead to tremulous, quavery speech; the voice has a trembling quality. This usually appears in later life.

Perhaps the most difficult part of having ET is the embarrassment which can lead some patients to withdraw from social activities. Anxiety also aggravates the disease.

The treatment of ET is difficult, but can be very

helpful. Stimulants like caffeine should be avoided. Anti-PD medications are not effective. Your doctor may prescribe one of the beta blocker drugs, such as propranalol (Inderal)—unless you have asthma or certain heart problems—certain tranquilizers and physical therapy. Primidone (Mysoline) is often the first choice of neurologists, followed by propranolol (Inderal). Deep Brain Stimulation is also very effective and is approved for use in ET by the FDA. It should not be used, however, unless the tremor is disabling and not responding to medications. With proper treatment these patients can enjoy life again.

For more information contact: **International Tremor Foundation** (ITF), 7046 West 105th Street, Overland Park, Kansas 66212-1803. Telephone: 913-341-3880. 888-387-3667. Fax: 913-341-1296. Web site: www.essentialtremor.org

References:

Larsen, T. A., Caline, D. B., 1993. "Essential Tremor." *Clinical Neuropharmacology.* 6:185-206

Koller, W. C., Busenbark, K., Gray, C. et al. 1992. "Classification of Essential Tremor." *Clinical Neuropharmacology.* 15:81-87

3

Parkinson's Disease and Heredity

Until rather recently, most neurologists were convinced that heredity played a minor role in PD. There were a few rare families with multiple members having PD, but nothing convincing for a hereditary cause in the many cases worldwide. New discoveries in the past few years refute these earlier notions and suggest that in patients with early onset disease, heredity may play a role. Nevertheless, familial PD is rare. Many cases previously reported as PD were actually ET. This is why a proper neurological examination is so important.

Questions about heredity in PD are frequent. Again, I will give you a sample of the questions asked, followed by my answer.

Question:

- *My grandmother had PD and I have noticed that I am beginning to get a slight tremor in my hands. Is there any evidence that PD is hereditary?*

- *Both of my parents have PD. My dad's mom's sister also had it. What have you heard about heredity playing a role and what are the chances that I would get it with both parents having PD? I think I heard that there is a 10% chance if one parent has been diagnosed. Thank you.*

ANSWER:

Over the past few years there have been many new and exciting discoveries about heredity in PD. Early onset PD may have a positive family history, twin studies have given us new insight into the genetics of the disease, and environmental toxins, plus hereditary factors, may indeed play a role in causing PD. The following is an up-to-date review of what is known.

WHAT HAVE WE LEARNED SO FAR?

Based on new compelling evidence, it now appears that PD involves both environmental and genetic factors. Some cases of PD are primarily genetic with an abnormal gene identified. In other cases the disease appears to be clearly secondary to toxins such as that seen after MPTP exposure. MPTP (a heroin derivative) can cause a Parkinson's disease-like illness in man and animals, and has a chemical structure similar to many pesticides used in agriculture.

Perhaps of equal importance is the recognition that some cases of PD may have both heredity and environment as the cause. In fact, some scientists are beginning to speculate that PD may prove to be more than one disease or relate to several different causes, such as a genetic susceptibility, plus exposure to an environmental toxin. However, apart from the Parkinsonism observed after medications, cardiovascular disease, trauma to the head, post-encephalitic and obvious toxic chemical exposures, we still do not know the exact cause of PD in the vast majority of patients. The importance of genetics in most cases is unclear.

One very important discovery is that of a disease gene in a large PD family that originally came from Italy. The report appears in the June 27, 2000 issue of the journal *Science*. This finding was the work of scientists at the National Human Genome Research Institute of the National Institutes of Health. In the abnormal version of the gene, the researchers found a mutation in a single base pair—one incorrect letter in a string of more than four hundred that compose the instructions for making the alpha-synuclein protein.

These researchers suspect that the abnormal gene is responsible for a significant portion of PD with onset generally before the age of sixty. Because the gene plays a role in the function of nerve cells, the finding also gives researchers a powerful new tool for understanding cellular abnormalities in PD. In addition, the finding of this gene will, in the future, serve as a clinical research tool within families especially prone to PD. It may permit new clinical studies looking for and investigating new drugs that could help postpone or protect patients from PD. Besides smarter drugs, scientists say that this finding could result in a better understanding of how PD evolves. The researchers go on to say that the identity of this gene also suggests an important new link between PD and Alzheimer's disease and may help in the development of ways to delay the death of cells (apoptosis) responsible for these degenerative brain diseases.

TWIN STUDY

In 1999 researchers at the PD Institute in Sunnyvale, California, reported on a study of 20,000 twin veterans of World War II, some of whom had developed PD. They studied both identical and fraternal sets of twins in whom one of the twins was known to have PD. They postulated that because identical twins share the same genetic profile, both members of these pairs should develop PD, if the disorder is genetically-based. They found that the second twin was indeed affected when the PD in the first twin began at an early age (before age fifty) confirming a genetic cause. By contrast, in the "typical" cases of PD (onset after age fifty), there was no significant difference in the incidence of PD between identical and fraternal twins (about 10 percent had developed PD). Their conclusions from the study were that early onset PD (before age fifty) is due to heredity, whereas the "typical" cases with onset after age fifty, are due to other unidentified factors, such as environmental toxins. They further stated that, with the differences noted between early onset PD and the typical late-onset form of the disease, the two may prove to be entirely separate conditions. This was an important study; but what about families with multiple members involved? Where do they fit into the scheme of things?

FAMILIES WITH PARKINSON'S DISEASE

In recent years, although still very rare, more and more families are being found with multiple members involved. In some of these families an abnormal gene has been identified. Why is it we don't see more of these types of families?

Most people with PD, when questioned, do not know of any affected relatives in their family. This may be partly due to the fact that this is a disease primarily of old age and many family members pass on before their PD shows itself. Some statistics reveal that half of all people with PD have their major onset of symptoms after age seventy-five. Adding to the confusion is that many times the symptoms of some family members are not typical of PD; others may have very mild symptoms that go undetected for years. Studies of these families have shown that affected relatives are nearly always concentrated on one side of the family, such as all on the maternal side (mother's side) or all on the paternal (father's side). Rarely are they found on both sides of the family. Also observed is that patients who have relatives with PD in the previous generation begin to manifest symptoms on an average of seventeen years earlier than their affected relatives.

It has been estimated that the risk of developing PD in the general population at large is 3 percent. Interesting is that people who suffer from chronic anxiety and depression have a likelihood risk of 6 percent, a connection for which there is no good explanation. In the United States alone there are probably ten million people at risk for PD. The chances of transmission of PD in familial cases is said to be between 10 and 15 percent. If both sides of a family (maternal and paternal) are involved, that figure rises to about 30 percent. The transmission of late-onset PD is thought to be in an autosomal dominant pattern. That means that each offspring of a parent with PD has a 50 percent chance of being a carrier of the defective gene. It should be emphasized that studies tend to show that only some siblings of the affected member are likely to ever experience symptoms of PD during their lifetime. This is thought to be because of a lack of what is called "complete penetrance" of the defective gene. It may also be that these uninvolved members are never exposed to some as yet unknown "trigger" factor that starts PD in motion.

The question might be asked here: "If I have PD and there are no other known family members with the disease, should I be concerned about passing the disease on to my children?" I believe most neurologists, based on present knowledge, would say the risk is very small; but with people living longer, no one yet knows this for sure.

GENETICS AND THE ENVIRONMENT

There appears to be a higher prevalence of PD in parts of the United States that are rural and agricultural. They include the Midwest, California, Florida and the Northwest. These states have a higher than normal use of fertilizers, fungicides, insecticides and pesticides— all of which could be implicated as a cause of PD. In fact, there is recent supporting evidence that certain common pesticides, may indeed cause a PD-like illness. In the December 15th, 2000 issue of the *Journal of Neuroscience* there is an article describing the "Combination of Pesticides Linked to Parkinson's Disease." This is the work of a team from the University of Rochester School of Medicine and Dentistry lead by Deborah Cory-Slechta, Ph.D., Professor of Environmental Medicine and Dean for Research. They studied the effects of a mixture of two common agrichemicals, the herbicide paraquat and the fungicide maneb. Each is used by farmers on millions of acres in the United States alone. Maneb is applied to potatoes, tomatoes, lettuce and corn. Paraquat is used on corn, soybeans, cotton, fruit and a variety of products.

In an experiment, mice were first exposed to either one of the pesticides alone. There were no significant findings. However when the mice were exposed to a mixture of the two pesticides, the animals developed all the hallmarks of PD as seen in humans.

An earlier study from Emory University also presented evidence that rats, when given a steady dose of the natural pesticide rotenone, used on home grown fruits and vegetables, also developed symptoms similar to those of Parkinson's disease. What is not known is how much of these pesticides remain on our foods once they reach the dinner table. The two pesticides are usually used at different stages of the growing cycle, but once these various treated foods reach the food chain, they both may be present.

This is the first time that outside pesticides have

been identified as possible environmental risk factors for Parkinson's disease. It is interesting that the PD-like effects on mice may be permanent, and that older mice may be more sensitive to the combination than younger mice. The team is also studying the effects of the mixture early in the life of the mice. Initial results have shown that mice with the same genetic abnormality, which causes some people to develop PD, are especially vulnerable to the mixture.

What may indeed prove to be true is that certain cases of typical, late-onset PD may also inherit either a genetically determined susceptibility to these toxins or some type of liver function disorder that affects their ability to detoxify certain chemicals. This may be a factor that influences their risk of developing PD. This could also account for the increase of cases in certain parts of the country.

References

Duvoison, R. C. 1996. "Recent Advances in the Genetics of Parkinson's Disease." *Advances in Neurology.* 69:33-40

Lazzarini, A. M., Meyers, R. H., and Zimmerman, T. R. 1994. "A Clinical Genetic Study of Parkinson's Disease-Evidence For Dominant Transmission" *Neurology.* 44:499-506

Wong, G. F. 1991. "Environmental Risk Factors in Siblings With Parkinson's Disease." *Archives of Neurology.* 48 (March):287-289

Semchuk, K. M., Love, E. J. 1993. "Parkinson's Disease: A Test of the Multifactorial Etiologic Hypothesis." *Neurology.* 43:1173-1180

Semchuck, K. M., Love, E. J., Lee, R. G.1992. "Parkinson's Disease and Exposure to Agricultural Work and Pesticide Chemicals." *Neurology.* 42:1328-1335

Tanner, C. M. 1999. "Parkinson's Disease in Twins." *Journal of the American Medical Association.* 281:341-346

Marder, K., Tang, M. X. 1996. "Risk of Parkinson's Disease Among First-Degree Relatives, A Community-Based Study." *Neurology.* 47:155-160

4

MEDICATIONS IN PARKINSON'S DISEASE

Prior to the introduction of levodopa the outlook for PD was grim. Patients suffered, their quality of life was poor, and for many their life span was significantly reduced. Then along came levodopa, which revolutionized the care of PD. Many patients could now lead more normal lives. But the benefits from levodopa proved limited and over the past few years new drugs like dopamine agonists and enzyme inhibitors have been introduced. Their addition has not only improved the care of PD but has prolonged the usefulness of levodopa, bringing new hope and comfort for PD patients.

Treating PD is somewhat analogous to treating diabetes. Treatment must be given daily, at precise times and for the rest of one's life. They do not represent a cure but they allow patients to lead more normal lives. PD medications are potent drugs that require careful dosing and medical supervision. In the pages that follow I will discuss one patient's problem, tips on taking your medications, drug interactions and drug-related Parkinsonism.

QUESTION:

Dear Doctor,

My father has Parkinson's disease. He is eighty years old. He has all the symptoms of PD. My first question is: "Are many people unable to benefit from Levodopa, and if so how do you know?" Secondly, my father takes this drug but has problems swallowing the pills, most of the time. Also, is there a good neurologist in my region of the country that I could take my father to for advice about his PD? His present doctor has not been helpful.

ANSWER:

Thank you, Jim, for your e-mail question regarding your dad. Most people with classic PD—those who exhibit typical signs and symptoms—respond when started on levodopa (Sinemet). However, in some this drug may only help the slowness of movement and the rigidity and only slightly improve the tremor, balance and other motor symptoms. Also about 15 percent of patients experience no benefit at all from levodopa. Most of these people have what is called "atypical PD." They have clinical symptoms that mimic the classic case of PD, but do not respond to levodopa. The way they have been clearly differentiated is by examining the brain at autopsy. These patients with "atypical PD" fail to show the diagnostic histology features of true PD: the characteristic loss of the dopamine-producing neurons in the substantia nigra.

I have two suggestions that may help your father. The Sinemet tablets should be taken one hour before or two hours after meals for maximum absorption in the gut. He should be on a regular schedule and the drugs must be taken exactly on time for each dose during the day. Secondly, with your father having difficulty swallowing the Sinemet, he can chew the tablets. This does not apply to the long-acting capsules or other medications. Sinemet tablets have very little taste and are well absorbed in the mouth.

As regards a neurologist in your area, I suggest you look at the resource section near the end of this book for the various PD Associations that you can contact for a referral. Ideally, you should try to find a neurologist who specializes in PD. Other good sources are local medical schools, PD research centers, and your state medical society.

TIPS ON TAKING MEDICATIONS

Just as people vary widely in PD symptoms and course, so do they vary in their response to drug treatment. There is no "one size fits all" treatment for PD. Some people do well with a particular drug, whereas others may not be able to take the drug at all—or they find that the drug does little to alleviate their symptoms. It is important to work closely with your doctor, letting him or her know how you are benefiting and tolerating your drugs in the dosage selected. By following your doctor's orders you should be able to find the right combination of medications that works best for you.

I would now like to share with you some tips I have learned over the years about taking medications. They include the following:

- PD drugs are usually introduced in low doses and gradually increased over a period of time. PD drugs often take several months to produce their full therapeutic effects so you need to be patient.

- Do not stop taking your medications or abruptly change the dosage without talking with your doctor first. Most PD medications need to be tapered off slowly to prevent undesirable side effects.

- Sometimes side effects are caused by other drugs you are taking for other medical conditions. In this case your entire drug regimen may need adjustment. And don't exclude over-the-counter herbal medicine, which you may not consider as medications. It is a myth that all herbal medicines are safe. They are, in fact, sometimes incompatible with prescribed medications.

- One of the most common side effects from PD drugs is nausea. For many, nausea is the reason a new drug is stopped, possibly prematurely. I experienced significant nausea from nearly all the PD medications I have taken. It should be emphasized that for most people, over time, this troublesome drug-induced side effect will lessen or disappear altogether. Again, try to be patient and don't discontinue the drug unless the nausea is unbearable or your doctor advises you to stop.

- To reduce the daily nausea, worse in the morning, I walked, took the drug with a glass of juice, and ate a few crackers. I finally found the best way to relieve my nausea promptly is crystallized ginger that I buy at a Peet's coffee outlet. One small slice is usually sufficient for relief. It is also available in many supermarkets. After several months my nausea from each new drug subsided and I was able to continue the medication as prescribed by my doctor.

- To achieve the best results from Sinemet (carbidopa/levodopa), take the drug at least one hour before or two hours after meals; in other words on an empty stomach. This increases the absorption of this medication. (Talk to your doctor about low protein meals and how this can affect how much levodopa gets to the brain). Absorption is also reduced by an acid stomach. If this occurs, chew an antacid tablet before taking the drug. Most of the other PD medications can be taken with meals and are not influenced by these other procedures.

- Take your medications precisely on time. Missing a dose by as little as fifteen to thirty minutes can result in a sudden "off" period which may last for hours. If you have missed a Sinemet dose by thirty minutes or less, chewing the tablets (tastes like chalk) can speed the benefits because of a more rapid absorption through the lining of the mouth. Do not chew Sinemet CR or any of the other drugs, unless so prescribed by your doctor.

- Don't try to make up for missed doses. If you missed a dose by an hour or more. don't double your dosage to try and make up. It will only increase side effects. Take your regular dose on time and get back on schedule.

- Carry your medications with you at all times and keep a few doses and a source of liquid in your car. If you get stuck in traffic, you will be able to take your medications on schedule.

- If at times you feel your condition is worsening, it can sometimes be due to another illness which tends to be masked by PD. PD can at times make you feel like you have the flu, so it can be confusing. Don't immediately ask to increase your dose of medication. Many times our sense of a deteriorating condition is temporary and disappears after a few days. If you increase your dose prematurely, you may find reducing the dose again difficult as the body may adjust to the increase.

- Drink lots of water. PD medications tend to dry out the body. Water—not juice, coffee or milk—helps kidney function and can flush out drug by-products. Water also keeps things moving by increasing bowel activity. Drinking lots of water helps relieve constipation. Unfortunately, our sense of thirst diminishes with age. Rather than wait until you are thirsty, drink water by the clock. Make sure you drink at least six to eight, eight-ounce glasses of water per day.

• Find a pharmacist who will keep track of all your medications and remain alert for dangerous drug interactions. If you are taking eldepryl (Selegeline), a MAO inhibitor, be particularly cautious of other medications, such as cold remedies and especially some of the selective serotonin reuptake inhibitors (SSRIs) like fluoxetine (Prozac), paroxetine (Paxil), and sertraline (Zoloft). Although interactions are rare when low doses of SSRI are used, many neurologists suggest that the eldepryl be stopped. Always read the label on the medicine and the package insert and if you have any concerns, contact your doctor or pharmacist before you take the medication.

• Keep a list of all your medications with the doses and time of day taken, in your wallet or purse. Give a copy to your spouse or caregiver, your doctors, and even to a friend or relative. Keep the list current. Join Medic Alert for a Medic Alert bracelet or chain which contains important information about you and becomes important in case of an emergency. (Call 800-432-5378)

• Read and learn as much as you can about your medications and their potential side effects. This may be lifesaving.

• Report any changes in your condition immediately to your doctor. Remember you are taking potent medicines.

• Comply with regular laboratory tests especially if you are taking Tolcapone (Tasmar).

• Although considered controversial by some, be alert for generic drugs that may not be as beneficial as the more expensive brand names. It is a misconception that generic drugs are all equally as potent as the brand name drug. A generic drug is essentially an imitation of an original brand-name drug. When the patent for the original drug expires, copies of the drug can be freely made. Many different companies may manufacture generics—meaning that many different versions of the drug may be sold at the same time. Some generic drugs, manufactured in foreign countries, may not come under the same quality control standards as the brand name drug produced in this country. Older patients may have a reduced ability to absorb drugs as a result of which their efficacy may be reduced. Consider this and discuss it with your doctor, if you think one of your generic medications is not working as well as expected. Generic drug substitution may not be the right choice for every patient. Problems that arise for patients are often due to a pharmacy's practice of switching patients from one generic to another generic manufactured by different companies. Thus, patients may experience dramatic fluctuations in potency and in some cases this can be clinically significant.

Don't be discouraged if you find a medication is not helping you or is causing side effects. Work closely with a neurologist who is willing to adjust your doses in a precise manner, so that side effects are reduced and your medicines act in concert to help relieve your symptoms.

DRUG-RELATED PARKINSONISM

QUESTION:

Dear Dr. Cram,

I am sixty-five years old, was injured at work, and strained my spine. I was given Flexeril and I developed tremors. At that point I was told I had PD. Can you get PD from taking Flexeril? It has been over a year since I stopped the drug, but the tremor at rest persists. I also have problems with my walking and speech. My father had PD.

ANSWER:

Dear Tom,

Thank you for your interesting question. Let's see if I can answer it satisfactorily. Parkinsonism can be caused by certain drugs taken for other conditions. Some drugs can produce a Parkinson's disease-like state that can fool the doctor and his patient until the drug is stopped. Other drugs make the PD patient's disease worse by interfering with levodopa function or interfering with receptor sites in the brain. These interactions can either cause serious side effects, or result in decreased efficacy of the anti-parkinson medications.

Drug-induced Parkinsonism (DIP), which is seen more commonly in elderly females, may be indistinguishable from PD, but there are certain clues. DIP is usually symmetrical at onset, unlike PD, which commonly begins on one side. Slowness seems to dominate the symptoms of DIP. A resting tremor and rigidity is less often observed in DIP. Adding to the confusion is that DIP may persist long after the offending drug has been stopped, subsiding after weeks or even months in some cases. If the symptoms have not gone in a year, then latent PD that is drug-induced is the likely diagnosis. In your case, Tom, Flexeril (cyclobenzaprine) is, to my knowledge, not a cause of DIP, although it can produce a tremor. However, with your father having had PD, plus all your other symptoms, chances are you may have had latent PD brought on by the introduction of Flexeril. An examination by a good neurologist would help. Time will tell if this is the correct opinion in your case.

The following outline highlights drugs that you should know about if you have PD. It is challenging to keep these lists current, due to ever-changing pharmaceutical advances. I offer this list as a place you can begin. Please be aware that up-to-date lists are also made available through the PD associations referenced in the resource section of this book.

There is no doubt that PD stands out as a disease requiring potent medications, many of which can interact with other medications and carry a high risk of serious problems—some of them life threatening. Prevention is only possible if the physician and the PD patient remain alert and question the possibility of a drug interaction before any new drug is started.

DRUGS THAT MAY INTERFERE WITH PARKINSON'S DISEASE

Some drugs prescribed for conditions other than PD may change or influence the brain's dopamine system. If a doctor prescribes any of the drugs listed below, be sure the doctor knows you have PD and is aware that the drug can alter your symptoms. In addition, be sure the doctor knows all the anti-Parkinson's drugs you are currently taking. Before taking any new medications, talk with the doctor about both the benefits and potential side effects.

In the following outline of potentially troublesome drugs, generic names are listed first; brand names are in parenthesis.

- **Anti-depressant Medications**

    Phenelzine (Nardil)
    Tranylcypromine (Parnate)
    Fluoxetine (Prozac)
    Sertraline (Zoloft)
    Paroxetine (Paxil)

- **Anti-psychotic Medications**

    Haloperidol (Haldol)
    Lithium (Lithobid-rare)
    Trifluoperazine (Stelazine)
    Chlorpromazine (Thorazine)

Perphenazine (Trilafon)

Thioridazine (Mellaril)—Low doses may be acceptable, but should be reviewed by your physician.

• **Anti-vomiting/Gastrointestinal Medications**

Prochlorperazine (Compazine)

Metoclopramide (Reglan)

• **Blood Pressure Medications**

Reserpine (Serpasil)

Rauwolfina Serpintina (Raudixin)

Alpha-methylodopa (Aldomet)

• **Post-Operative Medications**

Rescinnamine (Moderil)

Deserpine (Harmonyl)

DRUGS THAT CAN INTERACT WITH PARKINSON'S DISEASE MEDICATIONS

Drugs prescribed for other conditions may adversely interact with drugs commonly used to treat PD. There is some controversy in the literature that indicates the anti-depressant drugs, when used in PD patients, are tolerated well in low doses with few interactions reported. Even though reactions are rarely reported, doctors treating PD should evaluate each patient carefully before prescribing. If any of your doctors prescribes these drugs, let him or her know you are being treated for PD and what drugs you are taking.

Meperidine (Demerol)—Can interact adversely with Selegeline (Eldepryl)

Phenetizine (Nardil)

Tranyleypromine (Parnate)

Fluoxetine (Prozac)

Sertraline (Zoloft)

DRUGS THAT CAN PRODUCE PARKINSON'S DISEASE-LIKE SYMPTOMS

Parkinson's disease-like symptoms, which include tremor, rigidity, slowness, and postural instability, can occur secondary to some drugs. A neurologist can often distinguish these cases from true PD. Once the offending drug is stopped the symptoms gradually disappear. Doctors prescribing these drugs should be alert to drug-induced PD and be especially careful in prescribing them to the elderly. On rare occasions these drugs can unmask a true PD.

Haloperidol (Haldol)

Chlorpromazine (Thorazine)

Thioridazine (Mellaril)

Trifluoperazine (Stelazine)

Reserpine (Serpasil)

Alpha-Methylodopa (Aldomet)

Prochlorperazine (Compazine)

Verapamil (Calan)

Diltiazem (Cardizem)

References

Raiput, A. H., Rozdilsky, B., Hornykiewicz, O. et al. 1969. "Reversible Drug-Induced Parkinsonism." *Archives of Neurology.* 21:632-657

Gibb, W. R. G. 1988. "Accuracy in the Clinical Diagnosis of Parkinsonian Syndromes." *Postgraduate Medical Journal.* 64:345-351

Gershanik, O. 1994. "Drug-Induced Parkinsonism in the Aged." *Drugs and Aging.* 5:127-132

5

STRESS AND EXERCISE

THE ROLE OF STRESS IN PARKINSON'S DISEASE

QUESTION:

Dear Doctor Cram,

I was diagnosed six months ago with Parkinson's Disease (PD). I have an eighty-six year old mother with age-related dementia and a thirty-two year old daughter with marriage problems. Everyone still comes to me with their problems and I am finding the stress level in my life more than it used to be. Any suggestions other than I tell my daughter I no longer want to hear about her problems and, at her age, she should handle them herself?

ANSWER:

Thank you for your question, Arleen. It is very important that you keep your stress levels low, as chronic stress can be an aggravating factor for PD. What you suggest in being honest with your daughter is a step in the right direction. People often rise to the occasion when someone they love is hurting. It could be that an open sharing with your daughter about your changing physical condition, your fears, and your need to reduce stress levels, could give your daughter an opportunity to grow both as a person and in her relationship with you. Ask her to recognize your needs, support you, and she may begin to respond differently to you, as well as to the issues in her own life. Encourage all those around you to help you keep your stress down and not let them pile their problems on your shoulders. Be firm about this and don't feel guilty. I suggest you review the section in my book, *Understanding Parkinson's Disease*, about stress and methods you can use to reduce it. (See end of chapter for reference.) We can't avoid stress entirely, but we can learn to live more comfortably with it.

GOOD AND BAD STRESS

We are all subject to stress. It is a common denominator in all of our lives, difficult to impossible to avoid. It can sometimes improve our lives, such as the stress associated with taking on a wonderful new job or an exciting project, so called "good stress." Or, it can so overcome our mental equilibrium that we become agitated and depressed, so called "bad stress." Each of us handles stress differently and there are several ways of dealing with it that can reduce its impact. Allowing stress to get out of control and to continue unabated can have potentially serious consequences, such as the precipitation of a heart attack or aggravation of a disabling neurological disease such as Parkinson's Disease (PD).

THE EFFECTS OF STRESS

All of us who suffer from PD are well aware of the effects of bad stress on our disease. A severe stressor, such as loss of a loved one, can cause a sudden accentuation of symptoms and/or reduce the benefits of your medications. It can be a helpless and frightening experience, especially when the disease has been under good control. Should this severe stress continue for a significant period of time, it can result in a PD that might be more difficult to control. This is why the control of stress is so important in PD.

DOES STRESS CAUSE PARKINSON'S DISEASE?

While researchers have ruled out stress as a cause of PD, it can definitely trigger symptoms or magnify them, especially tremor and hypokinesias (slowness of movement). For some the source of this stress may not be so obvious and needs to be identified. Different things are stressful for different people. Once identified, the stress should be dealt with, the goal being to reduce as much as possible its negative impact on PD.

STRESS AND YOUR PARTNER

One major source of stress which can be difficult to deal with is that coming from a spouse or partner. A distressed partner can exacerbate symptoms by exposing the patient to negativity. Although a long-term illness may bring some couples closer together, it can also strain a marriage or long-term relationship to the breaking point. Your partner may not be able or willing to endure the realities of coping with such a permanent long-term illness. He or she may feel angry or resentful that major aspects of the relationship may change, including traditional roles; or the partner may become fearful and overprotective. In some instances the patient may fear abandonment. Professional counseling for either partner may be recommended.

Facing your partner's reactions can be one of the most difficult aspects of PD. You may already feel like a helpless victim of a permanent medical condition over which you have no control. A negative response from your partner only adds to these helpless feelings. It is very important that you do not let your partner's emotional responses aggravate your PD. As the patient, you need to deal with this problem head-on by keeping a positive, upbeat attitude and not letting anyone drag you into a negative emotional situation or into their depression. A positive attitude towards your disease is the most important self-help strategy you can use. It also helps if you inform your partner that one of the most important things they can do for you is to try and stay upbeat. Also urge them to help you deal with the daily stresses you face in your life. This allows you the emotional freedom you need to concentrate on coping with your disease.

It is equally important that you acknowledge the great impact your disease will have on the lives of your partner, spouse and family. You are going to need their support. By communicating, being supportive, giving your partner space, sharing your emotions, maintaining mutual respect, compromising, loving, and helping each other to cope, you will be practicing the essentials for any happy relationship.

COPING WITH FEAR

One common source of stress is fear of the unknown. How rapidly will my disease progress? How long will I be able to work? Will I become completely disabled and dependent? Will my life span be shortened? Unfortunately, no one can answer these kinds of questions about PD with any degree of accuracy. It becomes important then that you take one day at a time; try to enjoy each and every day while you still can. Don't dwell on the unknown. The future will take care of itself.

MANAGING STRESS

Reducing stress in PD is important and should be an integral part of the treatment regimen. Exercise, relaxation techniques, and a sense of humor are all recognized methods for reducing stress. If you want to learn more about relaxation techniques for stress I refer you to my book: *Understanding Parkinson's Disease*, pages 25-29.

References

Greene, S. M., Griffin, W. A. 1998. "Effects of Marital Quality on Signs of Parkinson's Disease During Patient-Spouse Interaction." *Psychiatry-Interpersonal and Biological Processes.* 61(1):35-45. New York: Guilford Publications, Inc.

Sapolsky, R. M. 1996. "Why is Stress Bad For Your Brain?" *Science.* 272:749-750

Chung, Wetal. 1995. "Behavioral Relaxation Training For Tremor Disorders in Older Adults." *Biofeedback and Self Regulation.* 29 (June):123-135

THE IMPORTANCE OF EXERCISE

In no disease is regular exercise more important than in PD. This includes:

• aerobic exercises (such as walking, swimming, and cycling)

• stretching exercises (such as yoga)

• strengthening exercises (like using weights)

• a very specialized form of movement exercises, designed to reduce stiffness and tremor, improve slowness of movement, help balance and walking and improve speech. These last methods appear in a new book by John Argue (see references) and are especially useful for people with advanced PD. I highly recommended this book.

Many people wrote to me about exercise as in the example that follows:

QUESTION:

I am a caregiver along with my husband. His father lives with us and has been a PD sufferer for quite a while. It is difficult to know how to encourage him to take daily exercise, as he thinks it of little value. He loves to work in the garden and does spend some time there, but in winter he does absolutely nothing. He takes his medications every two hours and if he is the least little bit off time, he will suffer through the day. I am anxiously looking forward to reading your book and I will pass it along to my father-in-law. Although he would never openly read it, he will privately. How do I get him to exercise more? Thank you for your consideration.

ANSWER:

Thank you, Martha, for your question. I hope my book will be helpful. As to exercise I am a strong proponent of this in PD. The longer your father-in-law avoids exercise, the harder it will be to get him on a daily regimen. Encourage his working in the garden and perhaps you could get him a treadmill or exercise bike for use in the winter. What about getting him a small dog that usually requires twice-a-day walks. I hope my few suggestions will prove helpful.

USE IT OR LOSE IT

We are all familiar with the old cliché: "Use it or lose it," referring primarily to exercising the moving parts of our body. And yet I wonder how many of us with PD fully realize its importance or take it seriously. I feel very strongly that regular daily exercise can keep one ambulatory and independent for a very long time.

FACTS ABOUT EXERCISE IN PARKINSON'S DISEASE

Regular exercise is one of the most important self-help strategies for coping with PD, but it is not easy. Even healthy people have difficulty getting and staying fit. Most people avoid exercise altogether or try a few sessions and quit. With PD the fatigue, limited movement, stiffness in muscles and ligaments, and sometimes even breathing difficulties, make exercise even less appealing.

Research and the experience of thousands of people with PD confirm that exercise is vitally important for maintaining optimum motor functions. A study conducted at Emory University School of Medicine demonstrated that routine aerobic exercise improves motor function in mild to moderately affected PD patients. The patients participating in the active treatment program underwent an exercise program similar to that used in cardiac rehabilitation. Each patient walked or ran for forty minutes three times a week for twelve weeks. The exercise pace was adjusted using the patient's cardiovascular response to a supervised protocol. The results were that at the end of the study the cardiovascular fitness in the exercise group had improved 37 percent. The scientists concluded that aerobic exercise in PD can be safe and that it improves both symptoms related to the PD disability, as well as the overall fitness of the person.

There is no doubt that the desire and ability to exercise is influenced by an individual's life-long and more recent exercise habits, degree of gait abnormality and respiratory limitations. In a separate study, patients with mild to moderate PD were studied using a cycle ergometer designed to determine the degree to which abnormalities in respiratory function and gait affect ability to exercise. The results were encouraging for PD patients who wonder how much exercise they should undertake and whether it is beneficial. They revealed that the exercise capacity of people with mild to moderate PD was comparable to normal values obtained from healthy controls. The results support the statement that people with PD should be encouraged to perform regular aerobic exercises to maintain exercise capacity despite the presence of abnormalities in respiratory function or gait. To this I would add stretching and strengthening exercises as part of the routine.

THE BENEFITS OF EXERCISE

Exercise will not stop PD, but it may slow its progress. In addition, it may improve your body strength so that you feel less disabled. It can also improve balance, help you overcome gait problems, improve your posture, strengthen particular muscles, and improve speech and swallowing.

Doctors believe that physical exercise may improve brain function by improving blood flow to this organ. It is also believed that exercise may stimulate the production of a chemical, brain-derived neurotrophic factor, that may help repair and prevent further brain damage. We also know, of course, that exercise releases endorphins, the body's own "feel good" chemicals from the brain.

Exercise can reduce your dose of medications, especially in early disease, or enhance their efficacy. Most importantly, a regular exercise program may help you to feel more in control and give you a sense of accomplishment.

Participating in a structured class or program also helps keep you connected to others so you feel less isolated. Exercise can keep your muscles fit and reduces muscle and joint injuries. In summary, a regular exercise program can help you:

- Improve muscle strength and body balance

- Maintain a good body weight

- Reduce gait problems; improve posture

- Decrease speech/swallowing problems

- Sleep better at night

- Reduce muscle and joint injuries

- Improve mood and help lift depression

- Reduce your dose of medications; enhance efficacy

- Feel more in control

- Slow down the progress of your disease

- Keep you independent for a longer period of time

- Achieve a sense of accomplishment

- Reduce feelings of isolation

A WORD ABOUT EXPECTATIONS

Your expectations from exercise should be realistic despite its many benefits. When you were well, you may have worked out and quickly noticed gains in muscle strength and cardiovascular endurance. Things are different with PD. Don't be discouraged if your muscle strength and endurance show slow and minor progress. It is because your PD is continuing to progress. Nevertheless, any exercise program is, at the very least, helping you to cope with the progressive symptoms, especially the most disabling ones. It is enough that the exercises are helping you maintain a better quality of life and a sense of control and accomplishment.

Remember to always check with your doctor or a physical therapist before starting an exercise program. It is never too late to start. Choose an exercise regimen that can easily fit your daily routine. It does no good if you choose an exercise plan that you don't have the time, place, or physical capacity to perform. Choose one that you can and will do consistently; one that you like. Many PD patients make a program of regular aerobic, stretching and strengthening exercises a priority in their treatment plan. Once you start, make it a daily part of your life and keep it going for as long as you can. Ask your physical therapist or a licensed exercise instructor to help you design your program.

References

Canning, et al. 1997. "Parkinson's Disease: An Investigation of Exercise Capacity, Respiratory Function and Gait." *Archives of Physical and Medical Rehabilitation.* 78:199-207

Cram, D. L., 1999. *Understanding Parkinson's Disease.* Omaha, NE: Addicus Books

"Aerobic Exercise Program Improves Symptoms of Parkinson's Disease." *Parkinson's Disease Update.* 1993. 31:143-144

Hurwitz, A. 1989. "The Benefits of a Home Exercise Regimen for Ambulatory Parkinson's Disease Patients." *Journal of Neuroscience Nursing.* 21:180-184

Argue, J. 2000. *Parkinson's Disease and the Art of Moving.* Oakland, CA : New Harbinger Publications

6

Preparing for Hospital

Question:

Dear Doctor,

My husband who is sixty-five has had PD for the past eight years. Last year he developed a complication from one of his medications and had to be hospitalized. He came close to dying. I stayed with him almost constantly and I was glad I did because I soon realized how errors can be made in the hospital. Don't get me wrong, the doctors and nurses who took care of my husband gave him wonderful care, but they were so busy with very sick people. As a result my husband's medications were often not given on time, causing difficult "off" times. Also my husband's voice is very low and difficult to understand so that he was unable to make his wishes known. That is where my presence was helpful. My question is: Don't you think people with PD should have someone to help them in the hospital like I did to be sure they are getting the best care?

ANSWER:

Dear Margaret,

Thank you for a most important question. The answer is yes; it is called an *advocate*. An advocate is described as "a person who pleads for or in behalf of another." If you asked most people, "Do you need an advocate when you visit your doctor or go into a hospital?" most would say no. Most people are not used to asking for this kind of personalized help. We think we can handle this area alone.

In reality, with today's managed care and the increased pressures placed on nurses and doctors, nearly everyone should have an advocate, especially if you need to be hospitalized. The person who can best act on your behalf is someone close to you who knows your condition. This may be a husband or wife, partner, friend, or a caregiver. It also helps if the advocate has some basic medical knowledge. The advocate needs to be aggressive, on top of things and be willing to question the decisions made in the care of the patient. The advocate should be prepared to address such questions as: Why are you doing this procedure? Does it have risks? What are the possible side effects? Are there other alternatives? Can we get another opinion?

THE IMPORTANCE OF AN ADVOCATE.

No medical condition in a hospital needs an advocate more than someone with Parkinson's Disease. They may not be able or willing to speak out for themselves and they need a lot of attention and specialized care. Their medication schedule is unique and requires precision dosing. Since people with PD are mostly over the age of fifty, the chances of having or developing another illness that may require hospitalization are high. They also can develop complications from their basic disease, as well as serious side effects from the potent medications used. It is helpful if people with this disease and their caregivers make some advanced preparations as listed below and know what to do should hospitalization be required:

- Make a legible list of your medications with doses and time of day you take each drug. Keep the list current.

- Because some hospital pharmacies may not stock certain medications, bring all your medications to the hospital in their original bottles to insure dosages are not missed.

- If an elective surgical procedure is to be performed, Eldepryl (Selegeline) should be stopped at least two weeks prior to surgery. This is because this medication can interact adversely with the pain medication, meperidine (Demerol). Also to be avoided because of potential drug interactions with Eldepryl are the gut motility drug metoclopramide (Reglan) and the anti-nausea drug perchlorperazine (Compazine). While observing the patient each day in the hospital, the advocate should remain alert to the possibility of a drug interaction or side effect when the patient's medical or mental status suddenly changes. The advocate should immediately inform the attending doctor of the changes. Drug reactions are more frequent in the elderly.

• Although this subject is disturbing, it is the responsibility of the patient and family to inform your doctors and the hospital after your admission, if you have a Living Will or Power of Attorney for Health Care. A Living Will is the statement of your desire to die with dignity and stresses the desire that no life-saving procedures are to be implemented when a terminal illness is reached. The Power of Attorney for Health Care identifies someone you trust—possibly your advocate—to act on your behalf, should you become incapacitated. It is a part of good planning that you have these sensitive legal documents prepared and in order before you enter the hospital.

• Support hose should be fitted on the legs to help prevent blood clots. The advocate may need to remind the nursing staff of this, as well as getting the patient to walk as much as possible. Leg and foot exercises by the patient in bed should be encouraged.

• One of the most important problems for the hospitalized PD patient is receiving their prescribed medications exactly as prescribed, in the correct dosages, and time intervals. Unless the attending physician is a neurologist or a doctor familiar with PD, errors in proper dispensing can occur. Doctors write hospital medications using Latin abbreviations such as TID (three times a day) or QID (four times a day) and all of the medicines are dispersed by the nurses at specific intervals during the day. People with PD, however, take their medications at various but precise times during the day and sometimes at night. These may not coincide with the scheduled times for nurses to make their medication rounds. The dosing times for PD patients have to be exact, as failure to do so can result in periods when the patient's disease is no longer in control, resulting in motor fluctuations with reduced mobility. On arrival at the hospital the advocate should present the patient medication list to the nurse in charge and explain why the drugs must be given at specific times. The advocate should also go over the list with the attending physician, who may not be familiar with some of the drugs used and their potential side effects.

As careful as they try to be, doctors and nurses can sometimes make mistakes. With the introduction of managed care, demands on nurses and physicians have increased and only the sickest patients are admitted to the hospital. This increases the importance of an advocate. The advocate, who is usually a spouse or family member, should try to establish some rapport with the attending physician and the nurses. This means the advocate should not act like a policeman, but more like a spokesperson for the patient—someone who asks questions and is looking out for the patient's interests when he or she is least able to do so. If the advocate is not happy with the way things are going and questions the quality of care, they should discuss their concerns with the medical staff. If things don't improve, they should consider changing doctors.

In discussing the advocacy subject with patients and medical personnel alike, there is general consensus that the advocate plays an important role in helping insure that the patient is getting the safest and the most effective treatments at all times during a hospital stay. If you or a loved one has PD, be prepared. Appoint someone now who you can trust will be a good advocate, should hospitalization become necessary.

7

PROBLEMS WITH VISION, SLEEP AND RESTLESS LEGS

VISUAL COMPLAINTS IN PARKINSON'S DISEASE

Visual complaints are not usually considered a clinical symptom of PD and yet vague visual disturbances are frequently reported. People so afflicted often complain of blurred vision. As a result they may undergo needless eye examinations and changes in their eyeglasses. Attempts are made to correct their visual acuity only to find that their corrected vision is normal and there is no obvious eye disorder. Several people wrote me with complaints similar to the following:

QUESTION:

Dear Doctor Cram,

I am sixty-two years old and have had PD for the past six years. I am slowly getting worse, especially my walking and stiffness. But my main complaint is my vision. It really bugs me. I find that I can't read the paper very well in the morning until about one hour after I take my medications for PD.

65

Reading seems more difficult and my eyes seem to tire more quickly. During the day my vision at times is blurry, but only for short periods of time. I have had my eyes checked at least three times by my eye doctor and he says my glasses don't need changing, as I am seeing 20/20. He can't find anything wrong with my eyes. Another eye specialist I went to found I had an infection in my eyelids which he called blepharitis. He gave me eyedrops which cleared up a film I kept having in my eyes. Can you tell me why my vision seems bad when the doctors say it is normal?

ANSWER:

Dear Brian,

Your eye complaints are not unusual. I have experienced similar symptoms. Learning more about what is happening can help take away some of your worry about your eyes. The following is a review of this subject.

Most of us take clear vision for granted. Yes, reduced vision is expected with advancing age, but an eye doctor can easily correct the complaint by prescribing a new correction in a prescription. In PD, the situation is different. Here, we are often dealing with a variety of eye symptoms such as blurring, dryness, and eye fatigue that seems exaggerated and responds poorly to the usual corrective procedures. Is there "more here than meets the eye?"

THE ROLE OF DRUGS

One of the most obvious causes of blurred vision in PD is that secondary to one of certain PD medications, especially anti-cholinergic medications. They include trihexphenidyl (Artane) and benztropine (Cogentin). This can be remedied by your doctor by decreasing the dose or discontinuing the responsible drug altogether. Check with your doctor about possible drug causes if your vision is blurred.

THE IMPORTANCE OF EYE MOVEMENTS

The movement of the eyes is a crucial part of normal vision. It is important for orientation to our surroundings, visual acuity, reading, and movement. Its function is controlled by the brain, which sends signals back and fourth automatically in a healthy individual. In PD, the inability of the eyes to move properly can add to disturbances in gait and motor control. (See chapter 8 for tricks in freezing).

The muscles of the eye are usually affected, especially in the more advanced cases, which is similar to PD's effect on the other muscles of the body. The eye muscles are stiff and may move in an irregular, jerky way. The eyes may have difficulty in the up and down and side to side movements When reading, the eyes simply don't move properly in scanning the page. This makes following the word sequences on a written page very difficult. Reading becomes a difficult task and the eye muscles, which are rigid, tend to tire easily. Some patients with PD give up reading because of this, which is not good. Giving up reading can be the start of a progressive isolation from the outside world.

Other eye movements that may be defective in PD and affect normal vision are:

Fast Eye Movement.
This is essential to bring peripheral images into alignment with the fovea—the most sensitive part of the eye for close inspection. The time between the appearance of the target and the start of the fast movement has been shown to be significantly delayed.

Slow, Smooth Pursuit Movement.
Following the Target. PD patients have a significant decrease in this movement.

Scanning.
This involves larger changes effected by gross movements of the eye in search for known targets.

It is thought that the blurred vision experienced by some PD patients may be due to these defective motor control mechanisms of the eyes.

CONTRAST SENSITIVITY

Contrast sensitivity is the ability of the eye to differentiate the smallest possible objects that can be measured easily. Some patients with PD have an impairment of visual perception. The image to the brain is of poor contrast. The significance and cause of this is unknown. Patients' contrast sensitivity scores improve when the patient is placed on Sinemet. Visual acuity, using the standard distance letters chart, has been found to be poor in PD patients when tested in low light intensity. This is a practical result of the reduced contrast sensitivity previously discussed. A selective loss of visual acuity at low light levels is seen in PD. Proper, fairly intense lighting becomes important for the visual acuity and reading comfort of many PD patients.

DOUBLE VISION

On rare occasions, a PD patient may experience double vision. This is due to the fact that both eyes are not looking at the same point at the same time. It can be due to ocular muscle weakness, greater in one eye than the other. This often accompanies fatigue and benefits from rest and proper doses of PD medications.

DOPAMINE IN THE RETINA

PD is not just a disease of the brain, but can involve the visual pathways as well. Various scientific studies have been done that reveal that PD does involve the retina of the eye. Animal studies using drug manipulations have revealed dopamine in the retina of the eye. A single human study demonstrated reduced dopamine content in the retina of a PD patient. Further studies of monkeys with MPTP (a heroin derivative) induced PD have also found a reduced dopamine content in the retina of these animals. It is now known that the retina of the human eye has special nerve cells that contain dopamine. These findings may help to explain my experience and that of others that it is often difficult to read the morning newspaper until the benefit of the morning levodopa dose kicks in. It could also help explain some of the subtle vision complaints of some PD patients.

The finding that the human retina contains cells that produce dopamine has some very important implications for brain transplantation research. Why these cells are in the retina and their function is not completely known, but they appear to be a potential source of dopamine-producing cells which until now have come from ethically controversial fetal tissue. In a preliminary study of seven monkeys with a drug-induced form of PD, inserting the retina cell implants into the monkey's brain resulted in an improvement in each animal of between 44 to 90 percent within three months. Titan Pharmaceuticals, Inc. has been leading this study. Their scientists believe that these retina-derived cells have a potential of "long-term," significant restoration of motor function, following their transplantation into the human brain. These cells have the advantage that they can be stored frozen and used as an off-the-shelf product.

The cells can be easily obtained from donor eyes at organ banks, grown and multiplied in the laboratory. For implantation, the cells are deposited on the surface of tiny gelatin spheres barely visible to the naked eye. Hundreds to thousands of these spheres, called

Spheramines, are injected into the brain.

One donor eye can provide enough cells to perform thousands of transplant operations on PD patients. Unlike fetal cells, these Spheramine cells are not attacked by immune cells in the brain, a very significant finding. Animal studies have so far shown "prominent" improvement in experimentally-produced disease. Human trials will begin soon. Although this work sounds very promising, it is too early to predict an eventual role of Spheramine in PD. The clinical trials will be carried out at Emory University School of Medicine.

In summary, these are some of the ways vision can be impaired in PD. Having difficulty seeing can be a most distressing symptom, and uncorrected, it can reduce the quality of life. Fortunately, levodopa replacement therapy can often help many of these unwelcome changes. But, just as with the primary disease, levodopa may become less effective in relieving vision problems in the later stages of this disease. More studies are needed on how PD affects our vision and attempts to find better ways to treat it.

References

Masson, G., Mestre, D., Blin, O., 1993. "Dopamine Modulation Of Visual Sensitivity in Man." *Fundamentals of Clinical Pharmacology.* 7(8):449-463

Vidailhet, M., 1994. "Eye Movements in

Parkinsonian Syndromes." *Annals of Neurology.*
35:420-426

Levin, B. E., Llabre, M. M., Ainsley, J., Sanchez-
Ramos, J. R. 1990. "Do Parkinsonians Exhibit
Visuospatial Deficits?" (Edited by Streifler, M. B.,
Korczyn, A. D., Melamed, E., Youdim, M. B. H.)
Advances in Neurology. 53:311-316 New York:
Raven Press

Duvoisin, R. C., Sage, 1996. *Parkinson's Disease. A
Guide For Patient and Family.* Philadelphia, New
York: Lippincott-Raven, 42-44

SLEEP DISORDERS IN PARKINSON'S DISEASE

QUESTION:

*I have had PD for seven years and I have a sleep
problem. I am averaging two or three hours sleep
at night and one hour in early afternoon. I have no
trouble falling asleep at night, but I then awake
after about two hours and have trouble getting
back to sleep. I then may sleep another hour or two
and I am up having breakfast at 4:30 or 5:00. Can
I expect any improvement without taking any specific medication? What steps should be taken to
that effect?*

ANSWER:

Thank you for your question about PD and a sleep
disorder, Norm. You are not alone. Between 75 to 95 percent of people with PD have some kind of sleep problem.

The effects of sleep deprivation on people with PD can be detrimental to their feeling of well-being to say the least. On the other hand, after a good night's sleep, many PD patients notice an improvement in their symptoms of PD. This is called "sleep benefit." It is thought to be due to a restoration of the levels of dopamine in nerve terminals during sleep. Sleep benefit tends to occur mainly in the earlier stages of the disease. I still experience it after eleven years with PD, but less than previously. When sleep benefit disappears, patients tend to experience motor fluctuations in response to levodopa. The loss of sleep benefit then often coincides with the appearance of gradual wearing off effects during the day. Napping during the day also helps reduce symptoms but, in my experience, only if the nap is at mid day (twelve to two PM) and no greater than thirty to forty-five minutes in duration; otherwise I feel groggy and uncomfortable on awakening.

The fragmented sleep in PD has been attributed to a number of factors:

- Increased skeletal muscle activity, disturbed breathing and drug-induced disruption of sleep patterns.

- Leg cramps, which are disease-induced, and nightmares, which can be caused by both the disease and the drugs.

- Dopamine agonists may cause daytime sleepiness as may PD itself.

- Depression, which is common in PD, can interrupt sleep.

- Fragmented sleep may be worsened by PD because the patient can't turn over easily in bed.

I myself have a problem of regularly awakening in the middle of the night, having difficulty getting back to sleep and averaging four to five hours a night with a twenty to thirty minute nap at noon. I have become used to this, and because I am retired, I do ok on this amount of sleep, not having to be well rested every day. For many, this marked reduction in the length of sleep is a big problem and not easy to solve.

You may hear or get suggestions from friends and other lay people about ways to address your sleeping problems, such as changing or discontinuing your medications. I would not suggest you do this as a way to solve your sleep problem, unless your doctor orders it. It is always best to rely on your physician for such advise. You have not given me your age or what medications you are taking. In general, the following are some medication-free strategies you can try:

- Sleep only as much as needed to feel refreshed.

- Use your bed only for sleeping and not as a place to watch TV.

- Try to arise every morning at the same time every day. This helps stabilize what is called your circadian cycle, your body's internal clock, that when set results in regular times of onset of sleep at night.

- A steady daily amount of exercise often helps sleep. However, try to schedule exercise early in the day, not close to your bedtime or it may keep you awake.

- Reduce noise and keep your bedroom at a comfortable temperature.

- Hunger can interfere with sleep at times. A light snack at bedtime may help. Drinks that contain milk also seem to improve sleep.

- Avoid caffeine after 12:00 noon. This includes soft drinks with caffeine.

- Alcohol of any kind at night should be avoided. At first it helps, but then causes fragmented sleep.

- Reduce liquids at night so that your sleep is not disturbed by bathroom breaks.

- If you become frustrated because you can't go back to sleep, try harder by keeping the lights out and staying quiet in bed. If you still can't fall asleep turn on the light and read a non-suspenseful novel up in a chair or watch a non-violent TV program until you feel sleepy again.

- Tobacco also can disturb sleep.

If these suggestions don't help, ask your doctor about one of the benzodiazepines to use sparingly and irregularly as a sleeping pill. Some also find that a change in medications, such as Sinemet CR at night or taking an extra dose of tablet Sinemet may help. Others do not. This should be approved by your doctor. Work with your doctor on this. Sleep problems are rarely cured, but they can be reduced in severity. I hope my practical suggestions will be of help to you.

References

Van Hilten, J. J., Weggeman, M., Vander Velde, E. A. et al. 1993. "Sleep, Excessive Daytime Sleepiness and Fatigue in Parkinson's Disease." *Journal of Neural Transmission.* (PD Sect) 5:235-244

Mouret, J. 1975. "Differences in Sleep in Patients with Parkinson's Disease." *Electroencephalography and Clinical Neurophysiology.* 38:653-657

Hogl, B. E., Gomez-Arevalo, Garcia S. et al. 1998. "A Clinical Pharmacologic and Polysomnographic Study of Sleep Benefit in Parkinson's Disease." *Neurology.* 50(5):1332-1339

RESTLESS LEGS SYNDROME

QUESTION:

Dear Dr. Cram,

I have been told I have PD. I have all of the usual symptoms and do reasonably well. I am also bothered by the restless legs syndrome. When it is active I am up most of the night waiting for the next episode to occur. My doctor has put me on Mirapex (pramipexole) which helps control it but does little for my PD. Do you have any suggestions?

ANSWER:

The restless legs syndrome (RLS), Arthur, is not unique to PD. It may affect as many as 15 percent of Americans. The cause in PD is unknown and it is not considered serious. Try to tell that to someone who can't sleep at night because of this problem. Since this is a frequent complaint from people with PD and seriously affects their well being, I will elaborate more on what we know about RLS and how it can be effectively treated.

Restless legs syndrome is a condition in which your legs feel extremely uncomfortable unless you move them. Because this discomfort most commonly occurs shortly before you go to bed, it may have something to do with that circadian internal clock I mentioned under sleeping problems. RLS can disrupt sleep, leading to daytime drowsiness. Let me describe the symptoms in more detail.

There is an urge to move the legs. Some describe it as a sensation of something crawling or moving in the legs, tickling them deep inside. Or some have a deep uncomfortable ache and have a need to rub or move the legs for relief. Moving the legs relieves the symptoms promptly, only to return seconds later. There is a definite worsening of the discomfort when lying down, especially when you are trying to fall asleep at night or just sitting still.

The incidence of RLS is higher in people over age sixty-five. Recognized causes are iron deficiency and pregnancy. Some cases have been due to diabetes, kidney problems or alcoholism. Stress may also play a role in some people.

There is a related condition called **periodic limb**

movements of sleep (PLMS), which causes you to suddenly extend and kick your legs in your sleep in lightening speed. The cause is unknown. It occurs more commonly in older people and is not serious, except that it can result in a restless night for your sleeping partner. Many of us have experienced this odd symptom and are relieved to learn it is benign and not a symptom of PD.

As to treatment for RLS, ask your neurologist how medications can help. The first choice is often carbidopa/levodopa just before going to bed. Others report good results from one of the dopamine agonists like Mirapex or Requip. Sometimes a hot soothing bath helps. I had RLS which disappeared after I started on Mirapex. I hope this answers your questions and that you get the relief you seek.

References

Walters, A. S., for the International Restless Legs Syndrome Study Group. 1995. "Toward a Better Definition of Restless Legs Syndrome." *Moving Disorders*. 10:634-642

O'Keeffe, S. T. 1996. "Restless Legs Syndrome: A Review." *Archives of Internal Medicine*. 156:243-248.

Montplaisir, J., Lapierre, O., Warnes, H., Pelletier, G. 1992. "The Treatment of the Restless Leg Syndrome With or Without Periodic Leg Movements in Sleep." *Sleep*. 15:3912-3915

8

FEAR OF FALLING, FREEZING, AND LOW BLOOD PRESSURE

CAN FALLS BE PREVENTED IN PARKINSON'S DISEASE?

QUESTION:

Dear Doctor,

My mother has PD. She was on a cruise and did very well. When she got back, she started falling and took one last big fall (no broken bones or muscle breakdown). She has been unable to regain balance enough to walk unassisted, and needs a walker and one person to help her. She is extremely sensitive to medications, so she can't adjust either way. She is on PT and OT and is making very slow progress. Is this falling problem common? Do people regain their balance?

ANSWER:

Your question is a very important one, Roger, since falling is common in PD sufferers, especially in the later stages of the disease. What needs to be evaluated in your mother is what is causing her to fall. It is a scary problem for both the patient and the family, because it can result in broken bones or worse. I recently wrote an article about falling in PD. I've incorporated the content of that article below.

Postural instability and falls are common in PD and represent a major source of injury. In fact, falls from loss of postural stability is a major contributor to mortality in PD. Many patients are more disabled by their loss of stability on their feet than they are by any of the other complications associated with this difficult disease.

Even if no injury occurs, a fall may prompt the individual to further limit activity because of the deep-seated fear that they may fall again. This self-imposed reduction in activity is often the beginning of a downward spiral, which is all too common in PD. The paradox is that as activity is restricted in the hope of preventing falls, the risk of injury and falls increases due to the lack of exercise and daily physical activities. The possibility of injury from such a fall is also increased.

WHAT ARE THE CAUSES OF FALLS?

Factors like impaired vision, weakness, arthritis and dizziness can enhance the likelihood of a fall in anyone. Conditions that commonly contribute to falling include tripping over obstacles, non-level ground, unexpected shoving, and poor lighting. Although these conditions may cause anyone to fall, the following are reasons for falling that are unique to PD:

- **Freezing**. The feet suddenly stop moving and the person becomes immobile or frozen. This may last a few seconds to a few minutes and can frequently cause a fall. The cause of freezing is unknown and affects about 30 percent of people with PD.

- **Orthostatic hypotension**. A sudden decline of blood pressure on standing, resulting in light headedness and blurred vision, as blood temporarily leaves the brain. Unless one sits or lays down immediately, they may pass out and fall down, only to slowly recover as the blood pressure returns to a normal range. Both PD itself, as well as many PD medications, can cause this problem.

- **Dyskinesias**. Abnormal writhing-like movements of varying speed, most commonly involving the head, arms and upper trunk. These are often difficult to control with medications. When severe, they can cause a loss of balance and lead to frequent falls. Dyskinesias appear to be related to the prolonged use of levodopa, especially in higher doses.

- **The infirmity and frailty of advanced PD**. Too weak to stand without assistance.

Postural imbalance

As PD progresses, problems with mobility appear. The first and often the most important condition that causes balance problems as PD advances is postural instability. It tends to emerge ten or more years into the disease and usually progresses. Defined: "It is the feeling of unsteadiness while standing with the tendency to fall forward or backwards." The righting reflexes that normally help us maintain balance following an unexpected shift in weight are abnormal in PD. The affected individuals may find themselves walking forward in a series of small steps in an attempt to catch up with their center of gravity. This type of movement is called festination; it can result in a forward fall. (Festination can occur during freezing attacks as well.) Others may take hurried backward steps, so-called retropulsion, and fall backwards. The loss of postural reflexes often results in a fall like a statue. This is because of the person's inability to react in time to reach out a hand or make a corrective step to break the fall. Injuries from such a fall are often more severe and disabling.

Problems with balance in PD are frequently reflected in the person's posture. Their posture is often stooped and the body is bent forward. To compensate for the unsteady balance the legs are bent at the knees and the arms bent at the elbows. The knees are flexed to prevent falling forward. The individual may have difficulty turning while walking. The turn is often carried out in a number of small steps rather than as one smooth movement and a fall can result as the feet get intertwined.

Currently, not much is known about the underlying causes of postural instability or its therapy. It does not routinely respond to levodopa. In my own experience the early use of the dopamine agonist, Bromocriptine (Parlodel), seemed to help my balance, but I needed frequent increases in dosage and eventually developed side effects. With the introduction of the enzyme inhibitor, Tasmar (tolcapone), I have experienced better control of my postural instability.

Deep Brain Stimulation may also help the walking difficulties in some people, but often very slightly. Postural instability is an area of PD that urgently needs more study.

WHAT CAN BE DONE TO REDUCE FALLS?

More than eleven million people in this country over the age of sixty-five fall every year. Approximately one-third of patients with PD fall relatively frequently. Falls represent a real danger with a risk of bruises, and even worse, broken bones. A broken hip, even when repaired, can cause chronic pain and increased disability. Falling is also one of the major causes of death in PD.

The question asked in the subtitle of this article is "Can falls be prevented?" The answer is: not completely, but their number and severity can be significantly reduced. It depends largely on the following factors:

- Physical conditioning. People with PD should be on an exercise program as soon as the diagnosis is made. It should be aerobic to include walking, swimming, or a stationary bicycle and the exercises should be done consistently—preferably daily—for a regularly scheduled period of time. Maintaining your physical conditioning can be one of the best ways to prevent falls. This will insure that your legs stay strong, your gate and posture remain stable, injuries to muscles and tendons are prevented, and serious falls are reduced.

• As you grow older and become even less steady, continue even a modified exercise program and be alert as you perform more risky daily activities, such as climbing stairs, getting up too quickly, or moving too quickly. Don't run for the phone and don't let others hurry you. Ask for help when you need it and don't do something physical that is beyond your capabilities. Don't be self-conscience if you have to use a cane or a walker; they are your friends. Use common sense and good judgement. If possible, practice balancing exercises which you can learn from a physical therapist.

COMMON SENSE

These are some guidelines that can help you prevent falls:

• Avoid unnecessary drugs that sedate and slow you down.

• Allow a moment sitting on the edge of your bed before standing in the morning.

• Pay attention to each of your movements. Try not to do two things at once.

• Try to transform shuffling steps into a normal stride. Lift your feet as you walk and put your heel down first. Walk with a slightly wider stance and swing your arms to help your balance.

- When walking, avoid carrying anything in your hands—especially when using stairs.

- Always use the handrail provided, when you must use stairs.

- Avoid steep or slippery steps without assistance.

- Always take the elevator, if one is available.

- Do not walk in darkness. Use nightlights, preferably with sensors, strategically placed about the house.

- As stated above, use a cane or walker to help maintain your balance and avoid becoming too fatigued.

- Make walkways, stairs, and bathrooms safe.

- Eliminate loose rugs in your own home and avoid them when visiting elsewhere.

- Avoid shoes with high-grip soles and high heels.

- Learn how to fall by relaxing and rolling the head to protect it. Learn how to get up from a fall. A martial arts instructor or an exercise therapist can teach you this.

- Know your limitations and follow your instincts.

TRAINED DOGS

Dogs can be trained specifically for PD patients to help prevent falls, plus a number of other activities designed to help both the patient and a caregiver. In a PD walking dog program conducted at the neurology unit of the Pennsylvania Hospital in Philadelphia, they found that trained dogs could reduce the occurrence of falls by 75-80 percent. For example, if the PD patient stumbles to the right, the dog is trained to shift its entire weight to the left preventing a fall. If the person falls, the dog is trained to help them up.

When the PD patient stops walking because of "freezing," the dog is trained to put its paw on the top of the PD patient's foot For some unknown reason the freeze is broken and the patient continues to walk. These dogs not only reduce falls, but make wonderful pets, giving unconditional love. These dog training centers for PD patients are listed in the Resource section of this book.

References

"Falls in Elderly Have Multiple Causes." *Family Practice News.* 15 May 1992. p.54

Marshall, C. E. 1989. *Falls: A Serious Problem In Caring For The Parkinson Patient, A Practical Guide.* Edited by Thomas Hutton J. and Lynne Dipwl R. Buffalo, New York: Prometheus Books

FREEZING IN PARKINSON'S DISEASE

QUESTION:

Dear Dr. Cram,

My husband recently went through the "freezing" and had to stay out of work for two months. However, with an increase of his medications, the freezing has stopped and he has returned to work. Can you tell us more about freezing in PD? One more question and I will let you go. What is your opinion of support groups? I would like to find one so that I could have someone to talk to when I need it. My husband is not ready to go to a support group. I know he is afraid to hear something he does not want to hear. Dr Cram, thank you for any help you can give me on this problem.

ANSWER:

Thank you for your important questions, Marla. First, let me say something about support groups. I can't say enough good things about support groups. Apart from providing camaraderie and moral support, members in such groups can give you information about the latest treatments, referrals to physicians, and practical tips on how best to cope. Joining one of these groups with your husband will bring you into contact with others who are facing and coping with similar life challenges. There are many organizations to choose from: patient groups, caregiver groups, and groups for the entire family. Some PD support groups are targeted to specific ages like those for young-onset PD. Many people newly diagnosed with PD, resist joining a support group. They believe they can face their disease alone. They don't want to be associated with "sick people." That resistance often fades as they come to grips with their disease. A support group may help you and your loved ones to:

- understand more about PD and the physical limitations imposed by the disease;

- talk about your fears and concerns in a supportive environment;

- develop ways to deal with feelings like anger, quilt, and helplessness;

- stay motivated to use exercise and other self-help strategies to maintain the best quality of life possible; and

- learn more about the latest developments in PD research and treatment.

To locate a support group in your area see the resource section of this book for the Foundations you can call or write for this information.

I encourage you and your husband to go together. You need to face this problem together, so that you can better help each other. I am enclosing a copy of an article I recently wrote on my experience with freezing. The content of that article follows.

WHAT IS FREEZING AND
WHAT CAN BE DONE ABOUT IT?

It was a morning like any other. I rolled out of bed in my usual slow fashion, put my feet on the floor to begin to walk, and there it was; I could not move. My feet seemed stuck to the floor and the floor was not going to let go. In an attempt to overcome this weird event my body lurched forward but to no avail. I was glad I had something to grab onto, as I surely would have fallen in my attempt to walk.

Having written a book on PD, I knew immediately what was happening. I could now add "freezing" to my personal list of PD symptoms. Freezing is a sudden, temporary, involuntary inability to move one's legs and feet. It is as if someone hit an "off" switch and stopped you in your tracks. It occurs in about 30 percent of cases of PD, usually in the later stages of the disease. I was hoping I could avoid this symptom, because I also know there is no known treatment for freezing, although drug manipulation may help for a while. Once it starts, it usually persists occurring more and more frequently during the day. The episodes may also become longer and cause severe disability. Freezing is one of the major causes of dangerous falls in PD patients.

It is difficult to understand how quickly and without warning this new symptom appeared. One day my gait was normal and the next day I was experiencing a freezing attack. Nothing had changed and my medications had been working well.

It seemed like an eternity, but after a few seconds

my feet released from the floor. It was at that moment I experienced—for the first time—a second new symptom; I was "festinating." In Mosby's Medical Dictionary a festinating gait is defined as "a manner of walking in which a person's speed increases in an unconscious effort to 'catch up' with a displaced center of gravity." It is not unique to freezing attacks and can develop as a gait in people at any stage of the disease.

I suddenly felt propelled, up on the balls of my feet, charging in a series of tiny but rapid steps. After just a few steps, this new symptom also stopped as suddenly as it had appeared, and I resumed my normal gait. But it wasn't over. The whole process repeated itself several times that early morning, usually on or after making a body turn. The duration of each attack was a few seconds only.

Once my morning medications kicked in, the freezing episodes and festination stopped, which was a relief. Since that memorable day, however, the freezing has occurred every morning without fail. It also has appeared infrequently during the day and occasionally during the evening hours. I know it may never go away and I must learn to live with it. Just knowing what it is—and knowing more about it—helps relieve my anxiety. I hope this review might help you as well.

WHAT CAUSES FREEZING?

Freezing affects about one-third of patients with PD. It appears most frequently in those people whose disease starts with gait problems—unsteady gait, difficulty with balance, etc.—which is the way my disease started. This suggests that freezing may be caused by some brief but repetitive inability of the brain to transmit messages that control muscular function in the feet and legs. This may possibly be related to the prolonged use of levodopa. However, even untreated PD patients may have rare, brief episodes of freezing.

Freezing is uncommon in the initial two to five years of treatment for PD. It is in the later stages of the disease, after prolonged use of levodopa, that freezing episodes usually begin and tend to become more frequent and severe. The freezing episodes usually occur in a time frame of seconds and are unpredictable. The underlying theories as to the cause for this phenomenon are complex and are based largely on alterations of levodopa metabolism. A few of these theories are as follows:

- The formation of dopamine metabolites that act as false transmitters or as competitors against dopamine receptors.

- A reduction in the dopamine system's capacity to synthesize, take in, and store the dopamine taken in by the patient for treatment. A desensitizing of dopamine receptors has also been postulated.

- Changes in other neurotransmitter systems that control muscle function.

Questions that remain are:

❶ Is freezing somehow related to prolonged use of Sinemet?

91

❷   Why does it involve selectively the muscles of the feet and legs?

❸   Why are the attacks so brief in duration?

❹   Why do only certain PD patients get it?

At this time there are no answers to these questions. No one knows for sure what causes freezing.

TREATMENTS FOR FREEZING

Adjusting Medications

Actually freezing, or "start hesitation," as it has also been called, may be a manifestation of both inadequate or excessive dopamine. Adjustments in dosage of PD medications may help. In some patients, however, the freezing appears regardless of the medications and is resistant to any attempts to manipulate the dopaminergic dosage. These people experience freezing even while on optimal PD therapy. Their freezing episodes are the most difficult to manage.

If freezing occurs during peak levodopa levels, the patient may not be properly medicated and an adjustment in the dosages may help. If freezing occurs mainly during "off" periods then strategies that increase "on" time may be helpful. This may include dietary changes, such as reduced protein. Some neurologists have found that in "on" aggravated patients, discontinuing Selegiline (Eldepryl) alone can sometimes reduce the frequency of freezing episodes. These drug dosage manipulations are best done by an experienced neurologist. Do not make any dosage changes without the complete supervision of your neurologist.

What happens if medication changes prove unsuccessful? Is there anything else that can be done for this very troublesome and debilitating problem?

TRICKS AND OTHER SUGGESTIONS TO BREAK THE FREEZE

For some unknown reason people with PD tend to have freezing attacks when they approach a doorway, tight spaces, elevators, rows of chairs or pews, a doorsill, scatter rugs, steps, a curb, or when making a body turn, or merely crossing a street. Unless you develop a trick to get yourself moving again, you run the risk of losing your balance and falling. These tricks often involve sensory or mental imagery cues. The following are some of the known tricks that may help:

- Imagine a line or object on the floor in front of you and try to step over it.

- Walk over masking tape placed across a walkway.

- Hum rhythmic tunes or count in a marching cadence in preparing to walk through a doorway or to initiate walking.

- Have someone put their foot in front of you so you can step over it.

- Slowly rock from side to side to get moving again.

- Counting cadence to yourself, or aloud, when

you walk, may ease the process.

- Listen to music, especially marches, and march or imagine you are marching.

- Summon your willpower and take one long, firm step forward. Some believe, as I do, that this whole process is closely linked to mood and mental attitude. If I stop and concentrate on the muscles in my lower extremities, I can sometimes break the freeze and resume normal gait—a reminder of the mind-body connection.

- Finally, the most successful trick to overcome freezing for me I learned from John Argue. John, a true Renaissance man, is also an exercise teacher extraordinaire, who has written a "must read" book entitled: *Parkinson's Disease and the Art of Moving* (New Harbinger Publications, Inc., Oakland, California, 2000). In his book he emphasizes the fact that when you have PD, your movements, especially of your feet and legs, are no longer automatic and "we are condemned to a life of conscious actions." The trick he teaches for freezing attacks he calls mindful walking or "mindfullness." The important observation is that the problem lies in an impaired visual perception and in the brain, rather than in the legs. As for the eyes, the problem is "impaired coordination of the eye muscles" and the need for mindful measurements of the path you intend to traverse. As for the brain, "it cannot make its calculations until the eyes have first measured the distance of the path. The brain will not give the legs permission to move until it has made its own calculations." This entire process is totally automatic in a healthy individual.

The trick is easy and in my own experience works well every time:

First, estimate the distance in steps you wish to traverse to get to your chosen site, say a doorway. It does not have to be an exact measurement.

Say the distance out loud and as you start to walk count your steps out loud or hum a rhythmic tune that works equally well. Surprise, surprise! You will find you are now able to initiate walking, with the freezing gone—at least until the next attack. The more you practice, the easier it becomes, until it is almost automatic. Using this and the various other tricks reported above, you may find you have a way to be the master of this disturbing symptom rather than its victim. These conscious thoughts and movements will allow you to reach your goal with a nearly normal gait. For me this trick has been a revelation, but more importantly, it has relieved me of much of the fear, embarrassment, and burden that so frequently accompany a freezing attack.

Do surgical procedures help?

Pallidotomy does not help. Electrical stimulation, to include deep brain stimulation of the subthalamic nucleus, has been reported to help nearly all the symptoms of PD, with the exception of freezing.

OTHER METHODS TRIED FOR FREEZING

Treadmill exercise and daily walking can be helpful. This also helps keep the legs strong, which helps prevent falls.

A hand-held laser has been claimed to help overcome freezing. The patient is instructed to direct the beam to the floor in front of them and they step onto the point of light. Canes with modifications have been tried with minimal success.

Finally, dogs have been trained to help PD patients. This is discussed under the section on falling. Usually, at least one or more of these suggestions will prove helpful. I have also observed that a good night's sleep tends to reduce the severity of the freezing attacks the following day. Whatever you do, if you are having freezing, it is of utmost importance that you be vigilant and prepared at all times for a sudden attack that might catch you off guard and produce a potentially dangerous fall.

References

Ambani, L. M., Van Woert, M. H. 1973. "Start Hesitation: Side Effect of Long Term Levodopa Therapy." *New England Journal of Medicine.* 288:1113-1115

Fahn, S., 1989. "Adverse Effects of Levodopa in Parkinson's Disease." *Drugs for the Treatment of Parkinson's Disease.* Edited by Calne, D.B., Springer-Verlag, Berlin. 399-400

Argue, J. 2000. *Parkinson's Disease and the Art of Movement.* Oakland, California: New Harbinger Publications Inc.

ORTHOSTATIC HYPOTENSION IN PARKINSON'S DISEASE

QUESTION:

Dear Doctor Cram,

I have had PD for ten years now. I am on Sinemet 600 mgs a day, Eldepryl 10 mgs a day, Mirapex 2.5 mgs a day, and Tasmar 300 mgs a day. My liver tests have been normal. Up until recently I was doing fairly well. I am sixty-eight years old and use a cane as my walking can get a little off at times during the day. Just about six months ago I fell after my wife and I finished a heavy meal. When I stood up I immediate felt light-headed, my vision blurry and I fainted. Fortunately, I was not hurt, but I got scared. I went to my neurologist the next day. She checked me over and said I had orthostatic hypotension. She tried to reduce some of my medicines, but my PD got worse. She now has me use above-the-knee support hose which is helping. Can you tell me more about this condition and what more can be done. It scares me, because the attacks come on so suddenly.

ANSWER:

Another reason people with PD fall, Marc, is secondary to a sudden severe lowering of blood pressure on standing called orthostatic hyotension. Minor degrees of this often go unnoticed and require no treatment. However, when the standing blood pressure is no higher than eighty over fifty, symptoms will appear and active treatment is needed. The following is a review of this subject, which includes my personal experience.

One very troublesome new symptom for me that appeared about a year ago is orthostatic hypotension (OH). Simply defined, it is "a fall in blood pressure on standing." To better understand what happens in OH we need to know more about the nervous system.

THE AUTONOMIC NERVOUS SYSTEM

The nervous system is divided into several parts, one of which is the autonomic nervous system (ANS). It regulates the activity of the heart muscle, the smooth muscles of the gut and the function of our glands. It is further divided into two parts:

❶   The **sympathetic nervous system** which accelerates heart rate, constricts blood vessels and raises blood pressure.

❷   The **parasympathetic nervous system** which slows the heart rate, increases intestinal and gland activity, and relaxes body sphincters.

The ANS is therefore concerned with the control of the autonomic functions of the body, which include bladder, stomach, bowel, sexual function and regulation of blood pressure just to name a few. When this part of the nervous system functions abnormally, the symptoms are referred to as "non-motor"—not related to purposeful body activities. Other non-motor symptoms of PD are sleep disorders. As many as 70 to 80 percent of PD patients experience some type of ANS dysfunction.

For years, researchers have known that PD results from a loss of neurons that produce a nerve-signaling chemical called dopamine in one part of the brain. A new study reported in the September 5, 2000 edition of the *Annals of Internal Medicine* suggests that PD also affects nerve endings that produce a related chemical, norepinephrine, in the heart. Using a system called positron emission tomography (PET), researchers found that of twenty-nine PD patients studied, nearly all had decreased numbers of norepinephrine-producing nerve endings in the heart. This suggests that PD is more than a brain disease and may be caused by an abnormality that affects the peripheral ANS as well. Interestingly, many patients with a loss of norepinephrine-producing nerves throughout the heart also had orthostatic hypotension. They concluded that the loss of nerve terminals in the ANS may be the cause of the orthostatic hypotension in PD patients. People with a fully functional ANS are able to compensate for the decrease in blood output by the heart, because the heart responds by directing an increase in norepinephrine activity in the sympathetic nerves, causing blood vessel contraction. If the ANS is somehow damaged, however, this blood vessel and heart response does not occur and blood pressure decreases progressively, causing OH.

THE SYMPTOMS OF
ORTHOSTATIC HYPOTENSION

The body's blood pressure, which is usually measured by a physician or nurse, is obviously regulated by the heart and the blood vessel tone. Normally, the ANS acts on blood vessels to counter the effects of gravity allowing a uniform flow of blood to the brain. In cases of OH, this blood vessel tone is compromised, perhaps because of the new findings reported above, and on standing, blood pools in the legs. As a result the heart rate may increase and the blood pressure suddenly falls. This results in less oxygen-rich blood reaching the brain. If the blood pressure fall is severe enough, people with PD may experience a period of light-headedness, dizziness, unsteadiness, slowing of mental processes, blurred or even blacked-out vision, and fainting (syncope).

I have personally experienced a "pre-syncope" symptom, consisting of a sudden feeling of weakness and warmth in my head and upper body. This precedes the above symptoms by seconds, warning me that I must sit down immediately. You, too, may come to recognize your own signs of an impending attack of OH and learn to quickly respond accordingly.

To confirm the diagnosis the doctor or nurse takes the blood pressure first with the patient in a seated position and then on standing. If on standing the systolic (top reading) and diastolic (bottom reading) both fall significantly, the diagnosis of OH is confirmed.

WHAT ARE SOME OF THE RECOGNIZED CAUSES OF ORTHOSTATIC HYPOTENSION?

PD alone can be the cause of this symptom, but in typical forms of the disease, when the patient is not on therapy, this is uncommon. However, there is a rare, atypical form of parkinsonism known as the Shy-Drager syndrome, in which ANS dysfunction is a prominent feature. These patients may present with significant OH, bouts of syncope, impotence, urinary incontinence and impaired sweating, all of which may be severe and difficult to treat.

In the typical cases of PD, the most common precipitating cause is levodopa and other drugs used to treat the disease. OH tends to appear in some PD patients as their disease progresses and the dose of levodopa is increased. Add to this a dopamine agonist and/or an enzyme inhibitor and OH may suddenly appear. They are all causes of this symptom.

OH can come on after such simple things as sudden standing, or after other common events, such as climbing stairs, physical exertion, heavy meals, long periods of sitting, fatigue, heat and humidity, and after a hot bath or sauna. Untreated, it can be a very troublesome and even disabling symptom of PD. Just as with "freezing" discussed elsewhere, OH is another cause of dangerous falls. Older patients with severe OH, who suffer from frequent falls, may require around-the-clock nursing. Falls cause more injury-related deaths in the elderly than any other type of trauma.

HOW IS ORTHOSTATIC HYPOTENSION TREATED?

For minor symptoms of OH often nothing need be done. Or it may be successfully treated by such easy methods as maintaining adequate fluid intake and by increasing the ingestion of salt. For the patient who does not respond to these measures, the following more specific treatments may be helpful:

- Talk with your doctor about stopping any unnecessary medications. Nearly all anti-PD drugs may produce this side effect, so it may be difficult to stop any one of them, especially if they are helping your PD. A reduction in dosage is another option worth trying.

- Drink at least eight glasses of water each day and check with your doctor before increasing your salt intake. Don't increase it on your own.

- Try wearing waist-high elastic stockings to prevent the pooling of blood in the lower legs. Thigh-high stockings do not seem to work in most patients. They should be put on first thing in the morning. Let me warn you these stockings are difficult to get on. They require a great degree of pulling and tugging that may be physically impossible for some. You may need help. These stockings are uncomfortable in hot weather. In my experience, however, it was worth it, as they proved to be very beneficial. My OH attacks are less frequent now, but I still wear the elastic hose if I feel fatigued, am having dizzy spells, or plan to attend entertainment that requires long periods of sitting, such as dining out or the opera.

- Take your time when arising from a seated or lying position. Before getting out of bed in the morning, sit on the edge of the bed for a few moments before getting up.

- Have someone at your side when you stand up, especially after a long or heavy meal. Sit or lie down immediately, if you feel the symptoms coming on. It is also helpful, if you are physically able to do so, to sit down and put your head between your legs until the symptoms subside. Many PD patients can't do this.

- Keep the head of the bed elevated, or sleep using several pillows. This elevation of the head and upper body reduces sodium chloride (salt) loss from the kidneys during the night.

- For the more severe cases of OH there are at least two medications that may help. The first is midodrine (ProAmatine). This is a drug that produces constriction of blood vessels, causing increased blood pressure. Side effects are itching, tingling of the scalp, gastrointestinal complaints, headache, and dizziness. I tried this drug for a short period and had difficulty with urination. This may have been a reaction peculiar to me (idiosyncratic), but some patients, under the advice of their doctors, fare better.

- The second drug is fludrocortisone (Florinef). This is a synthetic hormone that controls the metabolism of sodium chloride (salt). It causes the kidneys to retain salt and raises the blood pressure. It has helped many refractory cases of OH.

As to my personal experience with OH, I still have a

few attacks each day, many of them brief, which I have quickly learned to recognize. By taking the immediate steps to prevent an oncoming episode—such as sitting down immediately or hanging onto something—I have had no falls. My present regimen is:

- increased salt and fluid intake

- keeping my head and upper torso elevated at night (very important)

- adequate rest

- being aware of the causes

- remaining vigilant for signs of an impending attack.

References

Goldstein, D. S., Holmes, C. L., Sheng-ting, B. et al. 2000. "Cardiac Sympathetic Denervation in Parkinson's Disease," *Annals of Internal Medicine.* 133/5 (5 September 2000): 338-347

Kaufman, H. 2000. "Primary Autonomic Failure; Three Clinical Presentations of One Disease." *Annals of Internal Medicine.* 133/5 (5 September 2000): 382-384

Hickler, R. B., Thompson, G. R. et al. 1959. "Successful Treatment of Orthostatic Hypotension With 9-alpha-fludrohydrocortisone." *New England Journal of Medicine.* 261:788-791

McTavish, D., Goa, K. L. 1989. "Midodrine: A Review of its Pharmacologic Properties and Therapeutic Use in Orthostatic Hypotension and Secondary Hypotensive Disorders." *Drugs.* 38:757-777

9

UNDESIRABLE SIDE EFFECTS

HALLUCINATIONS

QUESTION:

Dear Dr. Cram,

My mother, age sixty-five, was just diagnosed yesterday with PD. The doctor feels that her symptoms are "mild" at this time and has recommended she start on Requip (ropinirole) three times a day and slowly increased. He told her that all PD medications have the possible side effect of hallucinations. Now she does not want to take medications. She said that she would rather live with her tremor than have hallucinations. What is the probability of hallucinations? She has no signs of dementia or diminished mental capacity at this time. What form do the hallucinations take? How often? When? What are the implications of no medications? How do I convince her to try the medication? I know all patients are different, but any information would be much appreciated. Thank you.

ANSWER:

Dear Josie,

Thank you for your important questions regarding your mother's very recent diagnosis of PD. Your mother and the family all need some time to adjust to this scary development. Your mother, I am sure, is frightened and may now be a little confused on hearing the word hallucinations. The word itself can conjure up images of mental instability and loss of personal control. It is indeed true that approximately 10 percent of patients with PD, who are treated with medications, develop hallucinations. This number is thus small. However, approximately one-half of patients on levodopa for two years or more may manifest even occasional hallucinations. Some of these may also experience levodopa-induced dream disturbances.

Most hallucinations are visual. Typically, they are usually of people, animals, children or small adults. They tend to disappear when the patient tries to touch them. In other words, the definition of hallucinations is "the patient will see something when there is nothing there."

The hallucinations may also be auditory, usually of music or human voices, but these are uncommon and usually appear in the cognitively impaired. Hallucinations may appear once a day or several times a day and are rarely frightening once the patient knows what they are. Their frequency seems to be greater during evenings and at night. They are not a reason to delay or refuse therapy. If hallucinations occur, the medications can often be adjusted and the hallucinations subside.

The challenge of treating hallucinations is to be able to reduce the patient's anti-parkinson's medication enough to reduce or eliminate them, while at the same time keeping control of motor symptoms. If this can not be achieved, then the neurologist may have other medications to try to reduce this side effect.

Many neurologists now either hold off treatment of PD until the patient needs it; or they may start Requip or one of the other dopamine agonists. This is in the attempt to delay the introduction of levodopa for as long as possible, the goal being to possibly reduce levodopa side effects down the road. If a patient's symptoms are mild, there are no negative consequences to holding off on the introduction of medications. However, as time goes on your mother may need treatment to feel better and improve the quality of her life. With her doctor's approval, she should start on a daily exercise program which can further delay or reduce her need for medication. I also suggest you find a PD Support Group in your area and take your mother to the meetings. There, she can bring up her fear of taking drugs. I can assure you she will quickly learn that others in the group faced similar fears. With the help of the group her apprehensions will disappear and she will become more confident in her doctors and herself. Your mother's PD is starting at a time when a cure may be close at hand. As patients and families, many of us remain hopeful that new scientific breakthroughs will continue to be made to relieve symptoms and one day soon address the root causes of Parkinson's Disease.

References

Wilson, R. W., Tanner, C. M., Weingarten, P. A. et al. 1986. "Hallucinations in Parkinson's Disease." (abstract) *Neurology.* 36 (suppl 1):216

Tanner, C. M., Vogel, C., Goetz, C. G. et al. 1983. "Hallucinations in Parkinson's Disease: A Population Study" (abstract) *Annals of Neurology.* 14:136

Sweet, R. D., McDowell, F. H., et al. 1976. "Mental Symptoms in Parkinson's Disease During Chronic Treatment With Levodopa." *Neurology.* 26:305-310

DEMENTIA

QUESTION:

Dear Doctor,

My grandmother, who is eighty-seven, has developed a significant loss of her short-term memory over the last eight months. She has had PD for four years. Currently, she is in an acute care facility, undergoing physical and occupational therapy. We had a case management meeting and a nurse used the term "dementia." What is dementia and what can we expect to happen if this progresses? We are considering bringing her home to care for her and I need to evaluate if this is a viable option. Thanks.

ANSWER:

Thank you for your question, Heather. Dementia is the progressive loss of intellectual abilities and impaired memory to the degree that the person can no longer perform their usual duties. It is primarily a disease of old age occurring in 5 percent of people aged sixty or older and 30 percent in people aged ninety or over. The incidence of dementia in PD under age sixty is higher, with actual rates of between 15 to 30 percent. Alzheimer's disease is the most common type of dementia, but not all dementia in PD is Alzheimer's. The differentiation can at times be difficult.

Symptoms of all forms of dementia can be:

• loss of short term memory

• changes in personality

• impaired judgement

• loss of intellectual function

• restless wandering

• eventually the inability to perform simple tasks alone such as dressing and eating

• The person may eventually not recognize family or friends.

Unfortunately, there is no treatment for dementia, and the progression rate is variable. Because of your grandmother's advanced age, the symptoms may progress more rapidly. It would be nice if she could be cared for at home, but I would suggest you check out the alternatives soon. Your doctor and/or a social worker can help you here.

References

Brown, R. G., Marsden, C. D. 1984. "How Common is Dementia in Parkinson's Disease?" *The Lancet.* 56:1262-1265.

Lieberman, A., Dziatolowski, M., Kupersmith, M. et al. 1979. "Dementia in Parkinson's Disease." *Annals of Neurology.* 6:355-359.

Mayeux, R., Chen, J., Mirabello, E., et al. 1990. "An Estimate of the Incidence of Dementia in Idiopathic Parkinson's Disease." *Neurology.* 40N:1513-1517.

DYSKINESIAS AND DYSTONIA

QUESTION:

Dear Doctor Cram,

I am sixty-five and have had PD for six years now. I have begun to have strange writhing of my head and upper body, especially after my supper time dose of my medications. My neurologist suggested I reduce my Sinemet dose and cut my Mirapex dose by half. This helped reduce the movements but control of my motor symptoms is not as good. My doctor said I may have to choose between having a good gait or have the movements. I prefer the good gait. My doctor called the movements dyskinesias. He also used the word dystonias. What is the difference between these two and what causes them?

ANSWER:

Dear Ray,

Dyskinesias are troublesome involuntary movements that tend to be writhing in type. Dystonia are involuntary muscle contractions or spasms, producing abnormal postures and muscle cramps. They both may occur after being on levodopa for two to three years or longer—earlier in young-onset PD. They are a side effect of levodopa and are helped by adjusting the levodopa dose. The longer you are on levodopa the more likely these movements will occur. Patients receiving more than 600 mg per day of levodopa are also more likely to develop these motor complications. The movements can include jerks, nods, grimacing of the face, twitches or a feeling of restlessness often of the upper body. They can occur at peak doses or at times of wearing off. Dystonia can often appear in the morning called "early-morning dystonia" and often affects one foot with a painful cramp. Work with your neurologist to titrate your dosages to see if these abnormal movements can be controlled. Sometimes the patient has to decide between having the dyskinesias and having difficulty with their gait. Minor amounts of abnormal movement are usually acceptable for most patients. If the dyskinesias become severe enough gait and balance are affected to the point it can lead to falls. When severe and not controllable, deep brain stimulation or pallidotomy may be considered.

References

Mones, R. J., Elizan, T. S., Siegel, G. J. 1971. "Analysis of l-dopa Induced Dyskinesias in 51 Patients with Parkinsonism." *Journal of Neurosurgery and Psychiatry.* 34:668-673.

McHale, D. M., Sage, J. I., Sonsalla, P. K., et al. 1990. "Complex Dystonia of Parkinson's Disease: Clinical Features and Relation to Plasma Levodopa Profile." *Clinical Neuropharmacology.* 13:164-170.

Lost hope in Parkinson's Disease

Some of the e-mail sent me for help brought tears to my eyes. I would like to share one of these e-mails with you.

Question:

Dear Dr. Cram,

I am a social worker and I am, for the first time, working with someone living with PD. My role in this person's life is to help link him with resources that will help him purchase medication and remain independent. The gentleman was a very active and independent outdoorsman before the disease took over his life. He is currently sixty-five years old and was forced to retire some years ago due to PD. He is already very disabled, walking only with the assistance of crutches. He is now undergoing speech therapy, because he can barely speak. It seems that his disease is progressing rapidly. He is very proud and refuses to talk much about his PD. I think he has given up hope. Often when we are meeting, his eyes will well up in tears and he will appear to be very sad. I know that losing his independence is heartbreaking for him, yet he insists "that's life." He gives me the impression that his tears are only a physical symptom related to his PD. I want to refer him for counseling (support groups are out). My questions are:

- *Should I persist in trying to encourage counseling?*
- *Are the emotional reactions manifestations of the physical disease?*
- *How can I best be supportive?*
- *What literature can you recommend that will help me better understand PD? I would appreciate any guidance you can offer.*

ANSWER:

Dear Elizabeth,

What a challenge you have taken on and what a wonderful thing you are doing for this victim of PD. The challenge is to try and improve his speech, his physical health and his mental state. That will not be easy and will take time and willpower from everyone involved. Those of us with PD may face the possibility of a loss of several of our senses, to include speech and loss of smell and taste. Speech in particular is so important for our daily intercourse and without it we have no way to communicate. Some with PD speech difficulties retreat into a world of self-isolation and silence

Please consult my book: *Understanding Parkinson's Disease*, as I think it will help guide you in the right direction. Encourage your patient to read it or you read it to him. I think you will find it upbeat and may restore some hope to your patient. No one with PD should ever give up hope. We are so close to that cure and the introduction of new drugs which could help all of us. Let me address several of your concerns and list ways you can help. To answer one of your questions: Yes, people with PD tend to be more emotional and cry more easily out of both joy and sadness.

- First of all keep your patient as independent as possible. Urge him, with his doctor's permission and your supervision, to resume things he may have given up. Such things as being a part of a patient or neighborhood group, playing cards, etc. The goal of this is to try and help him to regain his self-confidence. When he is more in control of his life, he will feel less like a victim. Encourage him to do independent things.

- Focus on small victories and consider keeping a journal of these to review with him from time to time to boost his spirits.

- As far as the speech problem, 60 to 90 percent of people with PD have speech difficulties and some are severely debilitated by this. It is important to keep his speech therapy going. A good therapist can often help the patient devise ways to communicate, possibly by including a voice amplifier. Unless he continues to communicate, no matter how imperfectly, he could slip into a life of isolation and loneliness.

• Give him lots of encouragement and help him to maintain his dignity.

• Depression affects as many as 40 percent of people with PD. It is usually due to sadness, rather than guilt or self-blame. It may be due to depressed levels of serotonin in the brain. Sometimes, it is secondary to the PD medications, but this usually peaks in five to six weeks as the body adapts to the medication. Try to get him to a mental health specialist he likes. It may be he needs a select medication to help his depression. Tell him to arm himself with only positive thoughts.

• Despite the fact that he is using crutches, ask his doctor if he can start supervised daily yoga stretching exercises. This will help release those endorphins from his brain, which could make him feel better. Any kind of regular exercise can help depression, as well as reduce his physical disability, and it should be encouraged.

• We have not discussed his PD medications, but they should be reviewed regularly by a good neurologist to be sure your patient is taking the right combination. With the right medicines, his speech may even improve. I hope this patient will never become a victim of what I call "skillful neglect."

• Finally, work regularly with him and encourage

him. Treat him as you would a friend. And don't forget a bit of humor now and then—it can be the best medicine. Make his immediate surroundings pleasant and upbeat and **don't let him give up**. The best of luck.

Surgery in Parkinson's Disease

Deep brain stimulation

QUESTION:

Dear Doctor Cram,

I have had PD for over ten years now and I am sixty-eight years old. My PD, especially the past two years, has gotten worse and nothing seems to help my tremor or my balance. My medications are not working well and my doctor has tried me on several. I am becoming discouraged. I have been hearing about a new procedure, which is helping people like me, called deep brain stimulation. My doctor says it may be time for me to consider this. What do you think? Can you tell me more about it, and the risks? Thank you for your help.

ANSWER:

Thank you, Robert, for your important question about this new surgery for people with PD. Since the 1930s neurosurgery has been used to treat certain patients with advanced PD. After the discovery of anti-parkinson drugs, especially levodopa, neurosurgery became less common, because for most people the levodopa worked well in controlling symptoms. However, it soon became apparent that some people were not helped sufficiently with drugs, or the drugs over time were no longer effective. This rekindled new interest in surgical intervention. The earlier surgery, still done, but with technical refinements, uses a technique that destroys a tiny selected area of the brain responsible for the uncontrolled tremors or severe dyskinesias. These procedures are pallidotomy and thalamotomy.

Over the past few years newer and safer techniques for surgically treating the brain lesions of PD have been developed. One of the most exciting of these is Deep Brain Stimulation (DBS). The principle of this procedure is based on the observation that nerve cells, subjected to high-frequency electrical stimulation, are not able to work, but not permanently damaged as occurs in pallidotomy and thalamotomy. The final result is primarily the same, except that DBS does not destroy nerve cells and is a reversible and adjustable procedure. This means that if a new successful treatment comes along, the entire DBS apparatus can be removed with no harm done.

The procedure DBS, was discovered accidentally by the French surgeon Dr. A. Benabid, a pioneer in neurosurgery for movement disorders. The basic procedure consists of a wire surgically implanted deep within the brain and connected to a pulse generator, similar to a pacemaker, implanted near the collarbone.

Patients can activate the device by passing a hand-held magnet over the generator. The effects can be dramatic. Many patients who are shaking so uncontrollably that they can't hold a teacup begin to experience normal lives when the stimulating wire is placed in the thalamus. More recently, it has been shown that electricity applied to the subthalamic nucleus or globus pallidus can reduce tremors by more than 90 percent, and symptoms such as rigidity, bradykinesias, and dyskinesias by about 60 percent. At present there are three possible target sites in the brain for placing stimulating electrodes: the subthalamic nucleus (STN), the globus pallidus, and a subdivision of the thalamus known as Vim. All are performed through a small opening in the skull with the patient awake.

In order to prolong battery life, most patients turn off their stimulators at night. Currently, DBS of the thalamus is being used in other countries to treat essential tremor, PD, chronic pain, and dystonia. The FDA has approved DBS, but only for placement in the thalamus for refractory—difficult to manage—tremor of PD and for non-parkinsonian essential tremor.

Information, mostly coming from Europe, suggests that DBS can relieve other, more debilitating symptoms of PD, such as rigidity and bradykinesia. The benefits of DBS appear to last with continued use. In contrast is a 1997 report in the *New England Journal of Medicine* from a Toronto Hospital that cautioned that the surgical effects of pallidotomy seem to diminish after two years and the long-term effectiveness is still unknown.

The following kinds of patients are considered candidates for electrical stimulation of the thalamus. They include those who:

- Are unable to take anti-parkinson medications or whose medications are now ineffective for all symptoms, or are producing intolerable side effects.

- Have classic PD and must not be demented.

- Have a disabling tremor and have undergone one-sided (unilateral) thalamotomy.

- Have a severe tremor and want to avoid permanent invasive surgery.

- Have undergone a unilateral pallidotomy and do not want to risk a bilateral procedure. (Bilateral stimulation of the globus pallidus is possible with electrical stimulation).

As to which procedure to choose, you need to discuss that with your neurologist and neurosurgeon. If you are considering any of these surgeries, it is imperative that you thoroughly investigate the credentials of the surgeon. These procedures should be performed only by an experienced neurosurgeon, who uses microelectronic recording equipment, which can pinpoint the exact area of the brain to be lesioned or stimulated.

What are some of the risks and problems of DBS?

- A 2 percent risk of brain hemorrhage

- Problems with speech

- Stroke (rare)

- Infection (usually of the scalp)

- Abnormal movement, muscle contraction, visual flashes—all of which can be the result of improper placement of electrode

- Electrode breakage

- Need for battery replacement

- Also, some studies have shown a reduction of cognitive ability after DBS. Others refute that finding.

References

Cram, D. L. 1999. *Understanding Parkinson's Disease. A Self-Help Guide.* Omaha: Addicus Books, Inc. 68-74

Burton, T. M. 2001. "Doctors See Wider Uses for Neurological Pacemakers." *The Wall Street Journal.* (16 February 2001): B I and B 4

Kumar, R., Lozano, A. M., Kim, Y. J. et al. 1998. "Double-Blind Evaluation of Subthalamic Nucleus Deep Brain Stimulation In Advanced Parkinson's Disease." *Neurology.* 51(3):850-855

For more information contact:

Anne O'Sullivan, Administrator

NYU Center for the Study and Treatment of Movement Disorders

530 First Ave. New York, New York 10016

Phone: 212-263-1483

Fax: 212-263-8031

11

NEW DISCOVERIES

LOOKING FOR THE CURE

QUESTION:

Dear Dr Cram,

I am a PD patient anxious to keep up with the new developments, but I have a hard time finding them or even worse trying to understand them. Everybody talks about a cure, but from where do you think that cure will come? Will it be a pill, an injection, surgery or some kind of gene replacement method? I am confused. Can you answer my question in language I can understand? Thank you.

ANSWER:

Dear Daniel,

Those are good questions and they will not be easy to answer. I agree the literature about PD research is confusing and often uses very technical words. What I will attempt to do, is give you a concise overview of those areas of PD research that show the most promise. I will try to do it with as little jargon as possible. Understand, Daniel, that new discoveries are coming at a rapid pace, and a "cure" for PD may come from an area of science and study that we never expected. Major discoveries are sometimes serendipitous. Also, when we speak of a "cure," I believe many of us would admit that we would be happy with a treatment that could stabilize our disease at its present severity, with no further progression. I could learn to live with that. Ideal would be a treatment that relieves many of the major symptoms permanently.

With the heightened interest in PD a new optimism is emerging and with that comes the hope for a cure. Some are predicting that, if research into this disease continues at its present pace, PD may be preventable in the early 21st century. Let us hope they are right. The discovery of growth factors, stem cells, new genes, and surgical techniques, just to name a few, all hold promise of a cure. But defeating PD will most surely require new discoveries that no one can yet predict.

The areas of PD research that show the most promise are highlighted below:

- Neuroimmunophilins-Ligands

- Neurotrophic factors

- Neural tissue transplants

- Stem cell transplants

- Gene engineering and therapy

NEUROIMMUNOPHILINS-LIGANDS

This, in my opinion, is the most promising discovery of a potential cure for PD. Let me give you a short background sketch of how these compounds were discovered and how they appear to work.

The drug that started all this was FK-506, now known as Cyclosporine, an immuno-suppressant used to prevent rejection of organ transplants. It is also the first drug discovered which showed—in the test tube and in tissue—that it could stimulate the growth of brain cells and help partially rejuvenate nerves. Because cyclosporine is a powerful immune-suppressant, with troublesome side effects, scientists had to isolate just that portion of the drug that caused the benefit to the neurons and nerves.

They were, indeed, able to isolate drug-like molecules (called GPI-1046) that had these desired features and not the unwanted ones. When given to animals with PD-induced symptoms they were found to stimulate the re-growth of damaged neurons and eliminate all signs of PD. Another important feature is that these ligands can be given by mouth and cross the blood-brain barrier. A series of these ligands have now been synthesized. They bind to cellular proteins known as immunophilins, which are receptors on the cell surface that turn on repair genes within damaged nerve cells.

This growth factor, GPI-1046, when given to Rhesus monkeys with MPTP-induced PD, resulted in a dramatic improvement in symptoms. Monkeys with difficulty walking, climbing and feeding themselves regained these abilities. The brains of these monkeys under the microscope showed evidence of re-growth of dopamine nerve terminals. So far, in animal studies, no toxicity or side effects have been observed. These drugs can regenerate damaged nerves without affecting normal, healthy neurons.

In summary, these drugs work by regenerating damaged neurons, resulting in a more than 90 percent recovery of normal behavior in animal trials. The scientists hope to be able to reverse PD in humans through use of an orally active molecule that crosses the blood-brain barrier, which would be unprecedented. This could put PD patients back to normal function. This sounds like a potential cure? We await the results of clinical trials.

The two pharmaceutical companies, Amgen and Guilford, working together, have just completed a phase one safety study. Preliminary results appear to indicate these compounds are safe in humans but efficacy must await further clinical studies.

References

Joseph, P., Steiner, G. S., Hamilton, D. T. et al. 1997. "Neurotrophic Immunophilin Ligands Stimulate Structural and Functional Recovery In Neurodegenerative Animal Models." *Proceedings of the National Academy of Sciences.* 94:2019-2024

Neurotrophic factors

A substance called glial-derived neurotrophic factor (GDNF) was discovered in 1993. It was shown to promote the survival of neurons. What more do we know about this substance?

All cells, including nerve cells, self-destruct when no longer needed. This type of suicide cell death called apoptosis, is in the brain, under the control of a genetic program that is permanently "on." Unless these suicidal cells are given the message not to, they self-destruct. In the brain the survival signals that save these cells are called neurotrophic growth factors. It was first thought that these neurotrophic factors were only involved in early brain development, but it is now known they are also involved in the survival of adult neurons. This raised the obvious question, could neurotrophic factors help PD? Further studies have shown that these factors appear to not only slow the loss of nerve cells, but they may prevent further neuron cell suicide. This could result in a treatment that could slow or prevent the further march of PD.

Using a recombinant form of GDNF, Amgen has demonstrated in its laboratories, that r-metHuGDNF, which has to be injected into the brain, works to protect dopaminergic neurons against chemical insult and can ameliorate PD symptoms in chemically-lesioned animals.

The r-metHuGDNF, has been injected into the brains of Rhesus monkeys with MPTP induced PD. Significant improvement occurred in these primates as well, with a marked reduction of bradykinesia, rigidity, and postural instability. All the results indicate that GDNF may be of benefit in treating humans with PD. Perhaps the main drawback is that this molecule cannot be given by mouth, or injected into the blood stream nor does it cross the blood-brain barrier. It must be injected, once a month, directly into the ventricles of the brain through a surgically placed catheter. This study is ongoing at multiple PD centers in North America. So far, preliminary results in humans have not been encouraging.

References

Lin, L. H., Dohety, D. H., Lile, J. D. et al. 1993. "A Glial Cell Line-Derived Neurotrophic Factor For Midbrain Dopaminergic Neurons." *Science.* 260:1130-1132

Gash, D. M., Zhang, A., et al. 1996. "Functional Recovery in Parkinsonian Monkeys Treated With GDNF." *Nature.* 373:252-255

Lindsay, R. M. 1995. "Neuron Saving Schemes." *Nature.* 373:289-290

Steller, H., 1995. "Mechanisms and Genes of Cellular Suicide." *Science.* 267:1445-1449.

NEURAL TISSUE TRANSPLANTS

In the 1980s, neurosurgeons in Sweden and China transplanted tiny bits of aborted fetal brain tissue into the brains of PD patients. The idea was that if these cells "took," the PD patient would be able to produce more dopamine. However, success of this procedure has been slow in coming, hampered by ethical and moral issues. The controversy is over the use of human fetal tissue for the implants. Although a federal ban over this type of research was lifted in 1993, given the Bush administration's position on fetal tissue research, federal funding is not likely to be forthcoming in the near future. It appears that funds to continue this research will have to come from other sources.

Results released in 2001 from the first randomized, controlled clinical study of fetal implants for PD patients shows that the surgery helped a small number of PD patients, but not all who underwent the experimental therapy. The results were age-related. This was a study led by Dr. Curt Freed from the University of Colorado in Denver and Dr. Stanley Fahn of the Columbia-Presbyterian Medical Center in New York. Their study included forty patients with advanced PD present for an average of fourteen years. After one year the treated patients under age sixty (nine of the total) showed significant improvements in movement. Patients over age sixty who received the transplants, as well as the placebo group, showed no significant improvements. None of the patients in the study showed benefit from the therapy in terms of their normal daily activities. The implants also did not reduce the need for any drugs the patients were taking in the study.

The most shocking finding in the study was that in 15 percent of patients, the cells grew too well, resulting in too much dopamine produced in the transplant patient's brain. These patients developed as a side effect, uncontrollable writhing and jerking movements; dyskinesias of a severity never seen before. The scientists say there is no way to remove or deactivate these transplanted cells, so this nightmarish side effect may be permanent.

Although some scientists are eager to proceed, the results of this study, plus the dispute over ethical issues surrounding it, may mean that the grafting of human fetal tissue into the human brain may no longer be considered a safe, viable option for treating PD.

References

Freeman, T. B., Olanow, C. W., Hauser, R. A. et al. 1995. "Bilateral Fetal Nigral Transplantation into the Postcommissural Putamen in Parkinson's Disease." *Annals of Neurology.* 36:379-388

Freed, C. R., Green, P. E., Breeze, R. E. et al. 2001. "Transplantation of Embryonic Dopamine Neurons for Severe Parkinson's Disease." *New England Journal of Medicine.* 344:710-719

STEM CELL TRANSPLANTS

The discovery of the stem cell in 1998 has refocused attention to brain repair. Stem cells are the universal cells from which all cells are derived. They can be grown in test tubes and made to specialize into any type of cell, including neurons. Theoretically, if this proves true, PD patients would get an injection of these newly produced stem-cell derived neurons into their substantia nigra and be "cured." That sounds too good to be true, and considerable research remains to be done. There is also the issue of ethics as these stem cells come from human fetal sources. At the present time, the current use of human pluripotential stem cells is under discussion and remains an unresolved ethical controversy.

But scientists are resourceful. A recent study found that bone marrow cells can be induced to develop into brain cells. This gives scientists a safe, reliable source for stem cells. A recent discovery (April, 2001 issue *Tissue Engineering*) is the presence of adult stem cells in the human fat obtained from liposuction. The next step is to test if these cells will transplant successfully, transform into the right kind of cell, and prove to be as good as cells taken from a fetus.

Scientists at Lund University in Sweden have reported that human neural stem cells grown in the laboratory can be used to generate new neurons in the brain. The main limitations are safety and ethical issues. Alternative sources like the bone marrow are needed. Many are convinced, however, that in a matter of years it will be possible to use stem cells to repair damaged tissues and organs including the brain. This sounds like a potential "cure" for PD.

References

Thomson, J. A., Itskovitz-Eldor, J., Shipiro, S. et al. 1998. "Embrionic Stem Cell Lines Derived From Human Blastocytes." *Science.* 282:1145-1147

Gearhart, J. 1998. "New Potential for Human Embrionic Stem Cells." *Science.* 282:1061-1062

"Bone Marrow Cells Can Be Induced To Develop Into Brain Cells." In *Parkinson's Disease Update.* 2000 Issue 114:785-786

Barinaga. M. 1998. "New Leads to Brain Neuron Regeneration." *Science.* 282:1018-1019

GENE ENGINEERING AND THERAPY.

I have alluded to genetic engineering, whereby scientists modify the genetic code of individual cells to create dopamine-producing cells from other cells, even from skin cells. The implications for PD are obvious.

The other important area is gene therapy. The recent FDA approval of the first commercial use of gene therapy can open new ways in which this therapy can supply PD patients with the neurotransmitters they lack. People with hereditary diseases cannot make a certain protein because the gene that codes for it is damaged or missing. Gene therapy then is the implant of the normal gene into the body so that the normal protein will be generated. Although gene therapy sounds easy on paper, it actually is a difficult and complex procedure which must be methodically done.

The main concern is safety. In present techniques, a disabled virus is used to introduce genes into the cells. The risk is that the viral vector might trigger the wrong genes in the person's DNA or become active itself. The other major concern is possible severe side effects from the procedure that may be life-threatening.

A recent gene experiment from the Research Center for Brain Repair at the Rush Presbyterian-St. Lukes Medical Center in Chicago, using experimentally induced parkinsonism in monkeys, relieved the severe symptoms in these monkeys and restored them to normal. Gene therapy for PD sounds promising, but scientists remain cautiously optimistic.

References

Pollack, A. 1992. "Gene Therapy Gets The Go Ahead." *New York Times.* (14 February 1992)

Freese, A., Stern, N., Kaplitt, M. G. et al. 1996. "Prospects For Gene Therapy in Parkinson's Disease." *Movement Disorders.* 11:469-488

Horellou, H., Mallet, J. 1997. "Gene Therapy in Parkinson's Disease." *Molecular Neurology.* 15(2):241-256

So, you have just been diagnosed with PD!

I end with this personal question I received one year ago. My answer gives me the opportunity to share with you how I felt on first knowing I had PD and ways I think one should approach this new challenge.

QUESTION:

Dear Dr. Cram,

I am fifty-two and have just been diagnosed with PD. As you look back to your early stages, what would you have done differently? I don't want end up lamenting "I wish I had known then what I know now." Thank you.

ANSWER:

Dear Coleen,

Thank you for your personal question directed at me. I gladly respond as follows:

As I look back on those early days, I, of course, was scared and suffering from self-pity. I allowed no one to know that, because I had made a promise to myself after my diagnosis I would not be a complainer. When someone would ask me how I felt, my reply was always "I am fine"—which was a lie. I guess I wanted to demonstrate to others how tough I was (or was it denial?) and that was not really necessary. Of course, the diagnosis came as a shock and I needed time to adjust. Because I now had my medical practice for sale, I felt I had, for obvious reasons, to keep my diagnosis a secret until it was sold. I even kept it from close friends. As a result of my mysterious behavior, I almost lost several friends. I should have trusted them with my secret. Besides, I needed their help. Here are some of the things I recommend if you are discovered to have PD:

- Start as soon as you can to get your life in order—your job, your family and your business.

- Accept the changing roles with your spouse or partner.

- Start to prepare in your mind for the future. Ask yourself: what will I do as the disease progresses?

- Don't waste time. Time becomes very precious when you have PD. My greatest regret was that I wasted the first four years in denial and self-pity, when I should have gotten off my duff and contributed.

- Start an exercise program immediately and try to stay on it for as long as you can.

- Learn all you can about the disease. Don't, like

many people with PD, be afraid to learn the truth. Knowledge helps alleviate your fears, can help you to make better informed medical choices, and can keep you aware of new discoveries. Remember, having PD does not have to represent gloom and doom. Modern medicine has changed all that for most individuals.

• Choose the right neurologist for you—one you can talk to, one who knows a lot about PD, one who knows how to adjust your medications for best results.

• Stay at your job for as long as you can, but if you need to retire, get any traveling in early. You never know how you are going to feel even one year from now.

• Live as normally as you can; maintain your social life and cultivate new friends as well as your old. Friends can be very helpful. Accept their help graciously.

• Remain productive and try to contribute to society

• Avoid stress from wherever it comes. It only makes you feel worse and can aggravate your condition.

• Join a PD Support Group to learn all you can about how others have coped with PD. Do not avoid them because you feel you are not as bad off as you think some of them might be.

• Think about preparing a room in your home for your care should that time come. Nursing homes are not always the best choice.

- Create a new life for yourself and your family based on support, communication, mutual respect, compromising, loving and helping each other to cope.

- Keep a positive attitude and never give up hope.

Glossary

A

Advocate: A person who pleads for or on behalf of another.

Aerobic Exercise: Various sustained exercises designed to stimulate and strengthen the body and the heart.

Agonist: A chemical substance or drug capable of activating a receptor to induce a full or partial pharmacological response.

Agrichemicals: Pesticides, fungicides and other chemicals used in agriculture to kill pests.

Akinesia: A kind of muscular weakness or loss of motor function.

Autonomic Nervous System (ANS):   The system of nerves that involuntarily control the functions of blood vessels, the heart, the bowel and glands.

Anti-Parkinson's Drugs: Drugs used for treatment of PD.

Alzheimer's: A disease of the brain resulting in confusion, memory failure, disorientation, and total disability.

Apoptosis: A death of cells by shrinking and disappearing, thought to be the way neurons are lost in the brain.

Atenolol: A beta-adrenergic blocker drug effective in cases of essential tremor.

Autosomal Dominant: A pattern of inheritance transmitted by a dominant gene.

Autosomal Recessive: A pattern of inheritance in which the transmission of traits depends on the presence or absence of certain genes.

Alpha-Synuclein: A protein produced by the PD gene discovered in a family with PD.

Anxiety: Anticipation of impending danger usually accompanied by restlessness.

Axons: A long extension of a neuron which conducts nerve impulses and messages to other cells.

B

Bilateral: Affecting both sides of the body.

Beta CIT: An investigational drug that when used with a SPECT can determine the status of dopamine in brain neurons.

Biofeedback: A relaxation technique in which people are taught to control some unconscious body functions such as blood pressure and heart rate.

Blood Brain Barrier: Thickly packed cells in brain blood vessels that prevent many substances getting into the brain.

Bradykinesia: A gradual loss of spontaneous movement.

Bromocriptine (Parlodel): A dopamine antagonist drug used to treat PD.

C

Caregiver: Someone who provides care for another.

CAT Scan: A computerized x-ray machine needed for some neurosurgical procedures.

Confusion: A disturbed mental state in which the person can be confused, disoriented and lack clearness of thinking.

Corpus Striatum: A mass of gray matter deep in the brain thought to help regulate motor and sensory functions.

Cyclosporin: An immune suppressant used in organ transplantation and a harbinger of GPI-1046.

D

Deep Brain Stimulation (DBS): The electrical stimulation of specific sites in the brain used to reduce the symptoms of PD.

Debilitate: To make a person weak.

Demerol (Merperidine): A narcotic pain killer to be used with caution in people taking Selegeline (Eldepryl).

Dementia: A loss of intellectual abilities.

Dopamine: A chemical messenger in the brain that transmits impulses from one cell to another and is deficient in the brain of PD patients.

Dopamine Receptors: Sites in the brain which are activated by dopamine and dopamine agonist drugs.

Dopamine Agonist: Antiparkinson drugs that stimulate receptors in the brain and mimic the effects of dopamine.

Double Vision: Also called diplopia, this is a condition of vision in which a single object appears double.

Dysarthria: Difficult or poorly articulated speech.

Dyskinesias: Abnormal involuntary movements that can result from long term use of levodopa.

Dyshagia: Difficulty swallowing

Dystonia: Slow twisting involuntary movements associated with muscle contractions or spasms and are secondary to levodopa use.

E

Endorphins: A group of natural substances in the nervous system that are released in response to stress and exercise and act on the nervous system to reduce pain, making one feel better.

Environmental Toxins: Harmful substances in the environment that are being considered as possible causes of PD.

Enzyme Inhibitors: Drugs that block the enzymes that destroy levodopa and dopamine.

Essential Tremor (Familial tremor): A disease in which the tremor is brought out by movement of the affected part. May produce a characteristic movement of the head.

F

Fetal Tissue Neurons: Neurons of human fetal origin which, when placed in the brain of PD patients, if they survive, could replace neurons lost by disease.

Flexeril: A drug used for muscle spasm.

Fraternal: On the father's side.

Freezing: A temporary, involuntary inability to move your legs or feet.

G

GDNF (r-metHuGDNF): Neurotrophic factors that promote the survival of neurons.

Gait: Walking or ambulation.

Gene Therapy: A challenging method using genes to treat disease.

Generic drugs: Nonproprietary drugs that can be sold without a brand name.

Globus Pallidus: A part of the brain important to motor function.

GPI-1046: Drugs that regenerate damaged neurons, so called immunophilins or ligands.

H

Hallucinations: Seeing or hearing things that are not there.

Heroin: A morphine derivative that is a narcotic and addictive.

High Frequency Electrical Stimulation: A reversible procedure in which a particular part of the brain is temporarily stimulated by an electrical charge to reduce a symptom or side effect in PD.

HMO: Health Maintenance Organization.

Hypokinetic dysarthria: Slow, difficult, poorly articulated speech.

I

Idiosyncratic: Something unique to that person; not a typical response to treatment.

Incontinence: Inability to control bowel or bladder function resulting in spilling of fecal matter or urine.

Insidious: Proceeding inconspicuously but with grave effect.

Intention Tremor: Tremor coming on with movement.

J - K

L

Laboratory Grown Cells: Cells such as stem cells grown in the laboratory for treatment of disease.

Levodopa: The generic name for Sinemet, the most important drug in treating PD.

Liver Dysfunction: The liver is unable to function properly in some way.

Low Protein Meals: Meals with a reduced content of protein.

M

Maneb: A fungicide suspected of producing parkinson-like disease.

Maternal: On the mother's side of the family.

Meds: An abbreviation for medications.

Messenger: A cell or substance that transfers information about the brain.

Midodrin: A drug used in the treatment of orthostatic hypotension.

Mirapex: A dopamine agonist used in the treatment of PD.

Monomine Oxidase Inhibitors (MAO): A general term for a group of drugs that inhibit the enzyme that oxidizes or breaks down dopamine.

Motor Fluctuations: The complications from the treatment of PD affecting the ability to move or increase motor activity.

Motor System Disorder: A disease like PD that affects body movements.

MRI: Magnetic resonance imaging. New radiological imaging techniques for surgical procedures on the brain.

MPTP: The abbreviation for 1-methl-4-phenyl-1,2,3,6-tetrahydropyridine, a heroin derivative that can produce a Parkinson's like disease in man and animals.

N

Nausea: Being sick to one's stomach.

Neuron: A cell which is specialized to generate or carry information from one part of the brain to another.

Neuro-immunophilins-Ligands: An exciting newly discovered substance(s) that stimulate the growth of damaged brain cells and nerves and appears to cause growth of damaged neurons.

Neuroprotective Therapy: Drug therapy for PD that may protect brain neurons from damage or reduce the rate of destruction.

Neurotransmitters: Any of several chemical substances like dopamine and acetylcholine that transmit nerve impulses in the brain.

Nor-epinephrine: An adrenergic hormone that acts to increase blood pressure by vasoconstriction.

O

Occupational Therapist: One who is trained to work with patients by providing therapy utilizing useful and creative activities to facilitate psychological or physical rehabilitation.

On-Off Attacks: A change in the patient's condition with sometimes rapid fluctuations between uncontrolled movements and normal movement, often caused by taking levodopa.

Orthostatic Hypotension: A lowering of blood pressure on standing.

P

Paraquat: An herbicide that, when added to maneb, can

produce a PD-like disease in mice.

Paternal: On the father's side of the family.

Patient Advocate: Someone who acts on your behalf when you are unable or unwilling to do so.

Pallidotomy: The surgical destruction of a small portion of the globus pallidus for the treatment of PD.

Parkinsonism: The combination of tremor, slowness, rigidity and loss of balance.

Parkin gene: The gene discovered in young forms of PD.

Parkinson Plus: Diseases that mimic PD.

Physical Therapist: One who has specialized training to work with patients to help them regain strength, coordination, balance, walking and endurance.

Postural instability: Impaired balance and coordination, often causing patients to fall backwards or forwards.

Propranolol: A beta-blocker drug used to treat essential tremor.

Q

R

Receptors: Sites in the brain that allow the attachment of certain drugs making them active and able to produce the desired result

Resting Tremor: Tremor of the limbs or body while at rest.

Restless Legs Syndrome: An uncomfortable feeling in

the legs, worse at night

Retina: The back of the eye that receives images

Rigidity: A symptom of PD in which the muscles and joints feel stiff and display resistance to movement.

Ropinirole (Requip): A dopamine agonist for the treatment of PD

Rotenone: A natural pesticide that was recently discovered to produce a PD-like disease in rats

S

Selegiline (Eldepryl): An MAO inhibitor used for the treatment of PD

Serotonin: An amine that occurs in nerve tissue and blood vessels and functions as a transmitter.

Shy-Drager Syndrome: A rare atypical form PD with significant dysfunction of the autonomic nervous system.

Sleep Benefit: A reduction of PD symptoms after sleep, seen usually in early disease

Social Worker: One who has specialized training to help improve social conditions in the community for people in need of this type of help and advise

SPECT: Single-Photon Emission Computer Tomography used to measure dopamine levels in the brain.

Speech Therapist: One who has specialized training to work with patients to restore speech and help with swallowing problems.

Spheramine: A gelatin disc containing dopamine-producing neurons from the eye to use in potential brain transplants.

Stem Cells: A type of cell recently grown in the test tube that can generate into other human cells.

Stem Cell Therapy: Using stem cells to create cells like dopamine-producing neurons from other cells and injecting them into PD patients as a possible cure for PD.

Stressor: A stimulus causing stress.

Stroke: An abnormal neurological condition in which blood flow to a part of the brain is interrupted, causing brain damage and sometimes death.

Subthalamic Nucleous: A part of the deep brain that transmits messages to the globus pallidus.

Substantia nigra: A movement control center in the brain where loss of dopamine-producing cells triggers the onset of PD.

Support Group: A group of people who meet regularly to support or sustain one another by sharing ideas and problems affecting them in common.

T

Thalamus: A part of the brain that receives information from the basal ganglia that coordinates normal movement.

Thalamotomy: Surgical destruction of a group of cells in the thalamus to abolish tremor on the side of the body opposite the surgery.

Tolcapone (Tasmar): An enzyme inhibitor used to treat PD.

V

Ventricles: Cavities in the brain filled with spinal fluid.

Y

Yoga Exercises: A type of stretching exercise that is helpful in PD.

Young-Onset PD (YOPD): PD with onset before age 40.

RESOURCES

Many of these organizations offer publications, newsletters and referrals to health care professionals and support groups.

The American Parkinson Disease Association
1250 Hylan Boulevard, Suite 4B
Staten Island, NY 10305
718-981-8001
800-223-2732
Web site: http://www.apdaparkinson.com
Offers publications and referrals to healthcare professionals and support groups.
If you need information about how to find a neurologist in your area call: The American PD Referral Service: 800-223-2732. For the West Coast, call Susan Daniels: 877-610-2732.

Parkinson Disease Foundation
William Black Medical; Research Building
710 West 168th St.

New York, NY 10032
212-923-4700
800-457-6676
Web site: http://www.pdf.org

Parkinson Disease Foundation
833 West Washington Bld
Chicago, IL 60607
312-733-1893
Offers a newsletter, extensive reading list, exercise program for PD patients and caregivers

The National Parkinson Foundation, Inc.
1501 9th Ave—Bob Hope Road
Miami, FL 33136
305-547-666
800-327-4545
Web site:http.//www.parkinson.org
Informational booklets and a quarterly Parkinson Report. They also offer an outpatient facility in Miami

Young Parkinson's Support Group
APDA Young Parkinson's I*R Center
1041 Foxen Drive
Santa Maria,CA 93455
805-934-2216
800-223-9776
A statewide support network for people with YOPD. Monthly meetings and statewide meetings are held several times a year

California Advocates for Nursing Home Reform
1610 Bush St

San Francisco,CA 94109

415-474-5171

This non-profit organization is dedicated to improving conditions in nursing homes. They provide referrals to care facilities, pre-placement counseling, a consumer guide to nursing homes and a lawyer referral service

National Institute of Neurological Disorders and Stroke
P O Box 5801

Bethesda, MD 20824

www.ninds.nih.gov

Parkinson's Institute
1170 Morse Ave

Sunnyvale, CA 94089-1605

(408) 734-2800

Parkinson's Support Groups of America
11376 Cherry Hill Road, No 204

Beltsville, MD 20705

http://www.fda.gov/fdac/features/1998/498_pd.html

Independence Dogs, Inc.
146 State Line Road

Chadds Ford, PA 19317

610-358-5314

Provides specially trained dogs for people with PD

Canine Companions for Independence
National Headquarters, PO Box 446, Santa Rosa, CA 95402-0446;
800-572-2275
Website:www.caninecompanions.org

Fidos for Freedom, Inc.
PO Box 5508
Laurel, MD 20726
(410) 880 -4178
Web site:www.fidosforfreedom.org

ON-LINE RESOURCES

The Parkinson's Web
http://pdweb.mgh.harvard.edu

Support for Parkinson's Disease
http//neurosurgery.mgh.harvard.edu/pd-suprt.htm

Parkinson's Disease: Hope Research
National Institute of Neurological Disorders and Stroke
http://www.ninds.nih.gov/healinfo/disorder/parkinso/pd htr.htm

Medic-Alert Foundation International
P O Box 1009
Turlock, CA 95381
800-ID-ALERT
Medic-Alert bracelets for emergencies

WE MOVE (Worldwide Education and Awareness for Movement Disorders)

204 West 84th Street. New York, N.Y. 10024

Toll-free number: 1-800-437-MOV2

Email:wemove@wemove.org.

Web site:www.wemove.org.

A non-profit organization formed to educate health care professionals, patients, and the public about all movement disorders including PD. Offers resources, research information, group events, and publishes the *International Guide to Patient Support Group Organizations*, available through their organization's web site.

INDEX

ABOUT THE AUTHOR

Fulfilling a lifelong dream, in 1959 Dr. David Cram received his medical degree with honors from the University of Wisconsin Medical School, Madison, Wisconsin. From 1963 to 1966, he trained for his dermatology specialty at the Mayo Clinic, Rochester, Minnesota, where he earned a Master of Science in Dermatology.

Upon completion of his medical training, Dr. Cram was assigned to the United States Air Force Base Hospital in Lakenheath, England, where he became Chief of the Department of Medicine. During those formative years of what was to become a prestigious medical career, he received the Air Force Commendation Medal and rose to the rank of Lt. Colonel.

In 1971, Dr. Cram joined the staff of the University of California, San Francisco, where he became Chief of the Dermatology Clinic. There he served as teacher, lecturer, and research scientist. Dr. Cram wrote more than seventy-five scientific papers on a wide variety of subjects with a special interest in psoriasis. He is known for establishing the first Psoriasis Day Care Treatment Center in the United States and was considered an internationally recognized expert in this disease.

Dr. Cram left his academic career and opened a private practice in dermatology in 1986. To his dismay, in 1989 he was diagnosed with Parkinson's Disease. Given the physical implications of the disease, he retired prematurely in 1991 from the medical practice he loved. With growing resolve, he took on the personal challenges of Parkinson's Disease. Bringing his years of scholarship and medical experience to bear, he began an extensive search of the literature to learn all he could about PD.

A disease known for its limitations and isolating effects led Dr. Cram to widen his outreach to PD patients and their families through his web page at Age Net, where he maintains an "Ask the Doctor" column. In addition, he has become a prolific author, having in the past five years published four books, including two on Parkinson's Disease: this newest book, *Answers to Frequently Asked Questions in Parkinson's Disease* (Acorn Publishing, 2002) and *Understanding Parkinson's Disease: A Self-Help Guide* (Addicus Books, 1999). His other two books are *The Healing Touch: Keeping the Doctor-Patient Relationship Alive Under Managed Care* (Addicus Books, 1997) and *Coping with Psoriasis: A Patient's Guide to Treatment* (Addicus Books, 2000).

Dr. Cram's many awards include an appointment as Clinical Professor Emeritus by the University of California in 1991. More recently, in 2001 tribute was paid by colleagues and supporters through establishment of The David L. Cram, M.D. Fund for Parkinson's Disease Research at the University of California Medical School, San Francisco.

Acorn Publishing Featured Titles

Answers to Frequently Asked Questions in Parkinson's Disease:
A Resource Book for Patients and Families
David L. Cram, M.D.

Seeds of Hope: A Physician's Personal Triumph over Prostate Cancer
Michael A. Dorso, M.D.

MindBody Cancer Wellness: A Self-Help Stress Management Manual
Morry Edwards, Ph.D.

Before You ... There Was Me ...
Dorothy A. Geary, Breast Cancer Survivor/Artist

The Courage to Live: My Personal Journey with God.
A Kidney Patient's Story
Carmen Buelvas Critchlow, Kidney Patient / Advocate

The Pill Box: One Man's Hopeful Struggle to
Overcome Manic Depression
Bruce R. Patzer, M.A.

Under the Camouflage:
Revolving Wheels of Time Power a Mother-Daughter Relationship
Sheila Evans

Firestorm. A Novel
Eleanor Weber Griffitts

From Other Dimensions. A Novel
Eleanor Weber Griffitts

Scarlett on the Case: A Children's Mystery
Kathy Mancl; Illustrator: Dona Fischer

As Strong as the Wind, As Deep as a Canyon:
An Adventure Story for Girls
Marijo Grogan, M.S.W./C.S.W.

Ancient Ancestors with Modern Descendants
A Companion for Studies in European History and Genealogy
Ronald Wells, M.D.

Please send:

_____ copies of *Answers to Frequently Asked Questions in Parkinson's Disease: A Resource Book for Patients and Families* by David L. Cram, M.D. at $19.95 each.*

TOTAL: _____

MI residents, add $1.20 sales tax: _____

Shipping/Handling: _____
$4.00 for first book
$1.00 each additional book

TOTAL ENCLOSED: _____

Name: _____

Address: _____

City: _____ State: _____ Zip: _____

❑ Visa   ❑ MasterCard   ❑ Discover   ❑ American Express
Expiration Date: _____

Please send check, money order, or credit card information to:

Acorn Publishing
P.O. Box 84
Battle Creek, MI 49016-0084

Ordering options:

Call toll free: **877-700-2219**

Online at: **www.acornpublishing.com**

*This valuable health resource is available to hospitals, treatment centers, shops, and support groups at discounted rates. For information, please call our toll free number. or e-mail us: **answers@acornpublishing.com**